MW00932550

Copyright © 2017 Justine Brooks Froelker, Ever Upward,
    www.everupward.org.
All rights reserved. No portion of this book may be reproduced, stored in a retrieval system, or transmitted in any form or by any means – electronic, mechanical, photocopy, recording or any other – except for brief quotation in printed reviews without the prior written permission of the publisher.

Printed in the United States of America

@ *Let Our Faith Be Not Alone* by Robert Saey Band

@ 2014 Lindsey Henke, Still Standing magazine

@ 2010 *You Are More* by Tenth Avenue North

Scripture quotations (NIV) taken from
https://www.biblegateway.com.

Cover wrap photo: Ann Zamudio
        @2017 *Don't Talk About the Baby* – a documentary
Cover wrap design: Taylor Hiller
Cover, interior, everything: Chad Froelker

ISBN-13:
978-1544630663

ISBN-10:
1544630662

The Mother of Second Chances:
The Struggle Bus of Rewriting My Story of Infertility and Loss

by Justine Brooks Froelker

Acknowledgements

Thank you to my husband Chad; my business partner, my creative brainstorm partner, my rational sense of calm and my witness to my life. None of this would be possible without your support. I love you so much.

Thank you to my friends and family. It has been over three years filled with the support of shared blog posts, Amazon reviews and support in times of celebration and frustration of *Ever Upward*. I would have never stuck through this all without your support and love.

Thank you to my followers and readers. Thank you for allowing me the space to struggle authentically. Thank you for doing the work alongside me. And, thank you for the support of the blog and the book.

Thank you so much to Kelli White. Your eyes in proofing this book helped me so much in meeting my deadline. Your encouragement and support mean more than you will know. I am so thankful God brought you into my life.

To my fellow warriors in the infertility community, know that you can be okay, no matter what you get in this journey. Do this work with me and define your own happy ending. Thank you also for your support of me and of my work. Thank you, especially, for truly seeing me.

Part I: Year 1
Thriving and Not Just Surviving...2
Fear in Owning My Truth...4
Practice Happy...6
Embracing It to Truly Let It Go...8
Making Room for the Light...10
The Frankenstein Walk...12
Our Fellow Warriors...15
Wallow...18
Taking Off the Armor of my Choice...20
Lights in the Tunnel...22
We Hold the Pieces to Our Puzzle...25
My First Step Out of Rock Bottom...27
My Dementor...29
Chosen Children...31
The Childfree Mother...33
Mourning What Should Have Been...36
The Authentic Therapist...41
Almost Enough Moments...44
My True Witness of 30 Years...48
Celebrating to Embrace Jealousy...50
Scarred But Never Closed...53
Change the Why...55
The Complicated Gray...57
Not Just Another Birth Story...59
Seared Dates...62
Our Infertility Rap Sheets...65
Defining Our Enoughs and Everythings...68
A Thistle of Dichotomy...70
A Buried Treasure...72
Loss is Loss...74
Isaiah...76
When We Become a Mother or Father...77
A Letter to a Girl Trapped ...79
Choosing to Be Remade...82
An Imposter...84
The Most Ironic Story...87

Part II: Year 2
The Warm Embrace...92
Making It Well ...95
Out of the Ashes...97
Forever Changed, Never Fixed...99
Living in the Tension...101
Through the Darkness We Can Awaken...103
Moving Through Not Fitting In...105
My Christian Complexity...107
The Completeness of Just the Beginning...109
Shifting the Definition of Success...111
She Rears Her Brave Heart...114
Are They Thinking It Too...118
Or Just Stand...120
At Peace Is Not My Story Yet...123
The Accidental Farmer...126
Giving Ourselves Permission to Feel It All...127
The Post-It Miracle...129
Honoring Them...131
Hope...132
Birthing a Rare Kind of Parenthood...134
My Shifting Shadow...136
Mustered Grace...138
It Gets Different...139
They Count Too...140
Even In Our Longing...142
Negotiations with a Three Year Old...143

Part III: Year 3
Small and Mighty...145
The Empty Well...147
Identity Theft...148
Becoming a Gift...150
Loving Well and Fully...153
The Goosebumps of Knowing Awe...154
Seeing Me...158
A Strawberry Shortcake Bandage...160
The Permission of And...162
Four...164
A Story the World Isn't Ready For...166

Epilogue...169

Introduction

There are days I still can't believe my story is out there helping people. That my decently flawed light out of my own shit show of darkness has helped others shine their own light out of theirs. I wrote my first book, *Ever Upward*, because I had to. I was pissed at my choices for resources in the infertility and loss community. What I know now is that it was also the beginning of how I honor and mother my three babies every single day.

Three years ago I started the blog, simply in an attempt to get a publishing contract. Little did I know back then just how complicated that world of publishing is. The blog has taken on a heart of its own. It has connected me with the most incredible people from all over the world. And, it is as if is it's own Ever Upward story. As I am finishing up the follow up book to *Ever Upward*, *The Complicated Gray*, I knew I had to put out this very book you are holding in your hands for three reasons:

1. It deserves to be in print.
2. National Infertility Awareness Week needs more attention and stories like mine need to be a part of them.
3. And, I suppose a little income stream from writing doesn't hurt either, especially to keep what has become a ministry afloat.

And, so, here it is, over three years of raw, flawed and wholehearted writing from *Ever Upward* the blog. I have edited and updated some pieces a bit but for the most part they remain in their original text.

I hope you see the growth in my story, my truth and in my writing throughout the years.

As I prepare for *The Complicated Gray*, what I think is my most important work in this journey, to be released in the Fall of 2017, I hope this book helps you to do the work of this incredible wholehearted life.

To choose to define your own happy ending and to rise ever upward.

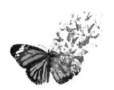

Part I

Year 1

Thriving Not Just Surviving

Every day I make sure to model to my clients the work I've done to change my life. And I am reminded that happiness is a choice we must make every day and that it doesn't come easily to anyone.

I've survived a year of my life in a body cast. Depression. The loss of 3 babies. The loss of my first furry child. The loss of future dreams. The loss of my identity and sense of belonging. And at times, the loss of my hope and faith.

I've had to redefine my happiness and choose to thrive many times over. And in the last year of my life, I've worked my ass off on becoming a better, happier and healthier person. And the more time that passes in this work, the more I realize that no one gets out of it. I honestly believe the people who are "making it look easy" aren't living the happy and fulfilled life they think they are.

Choosing happiness can be a huge pain and takes time, but it is also an effort that shows immediate payoff. I can stamp my foot and scream at the top of my lungs that this isn't fair. But the fact is, nothing in this life is necessarily fair or unfair. It just is. I can choose to focus on the uncontrollable or I can choose to realize the only real power I posses is what I do with the gifts, and the shit, that have been bestowed upon me.

That acceptance means I work every day, and sometimes every minute, to choose my happiness.

I thrive because…
I exercise.
I dance.
I listen to happy music.
I meditate.
I write.
I read.
I journal.
I eat right.
I help.
I engage and connect.
I live authentically vulnerable showing my soul to all the world.

I choose to continuously work on the art of letting go of what was never meant to be mine.

And I choose to embrace my whole self, losses and flaws, along with the joys.

And I choose, every day, to practice this happiness work and to model it to my clients. Showing them they aren't in this fight alone but rather have a knowing partner to walk alongside them, and at times push them forward from behind.

This journey has been a constant reminder that sometimes we just don't get what we wanted and that sometimes life just doesn't turn out the way it was "supposed" to. But that doesn't mean life hasn't happened exactly the way it was meant to. We just have to have the faith that we may one day get to understand it truly.

And in the meantime, I choose to embrace this uncertainty, trusting in my work and the practice of happiness.

As this is my thriving acceptance and my story, and therefore me.

Fearing in Owning My Truth

Three years ago it was a but or an either or scenario. Scary but freeing. Difficult but amazing. Sad but happy. Angry but accepting. Complicated but clear. Proving but owning.

What I've come to realize, with the help of my therapist (yes, great therapists have a great therapist, too), is I'm undeniably scared shitless of publicly owning my truth. Because even though it is my truth, it is also against the grain, misunderstood, and not considered the norm. This fear, if coupled with my innate calling to tell my truth, to own it and speak out, to live my authentic soul and to love my true calling, can create mind numbing, gut wrenching, and discontented paralysis. And bottom line, I never have, nor will I ever start, to live my life shying away from my truth.

So, here we go, the first post in truly owning my truth...

~ We stopped IVF before it worked. We stopped the hormones, the drugs, the painful procedures and the exorbitant amounts of money *before* we got a baby.

~ We are not choosing adoption.

~ And I'm okay with these decisions, I trust them, and I know they are right for us.

IVF can work. And it does work for so many. But for some of us, it just doesn't. Some recent reports state a 70% failure rate. We have to start acknowledging (and talking about) the whole story of IVF, the beautiful, healthy babies and complete families that can result but also the painful procedures, the risks, the money and the strain on our emotions, relationships, health, and the fact, that sometimes it just does not work.

Because when we acknowledge the whole story, we make room for everyone, even those of us who made an impossible decision to say enough is enough. Those of us who are working, every minute, to accept what was never meant to be and what is.

"Why don't you just adopt?" I know the words come from a place of love, curiosity and just wanting to "fix" my pain. But these words, more often than not, feel invalidating and minimizing. Invalidating to the journey we've been through with IVF, the loss of our 3 babies and our 3 dreams. And minimizing to the difficult adoption process. Adoption isn't for everyone, and I know that's okay, but also beyond terrifying to admit out loud, let alone here in print.

We are the only ones to make these decisions, for it is our family. We must make them because we know they are right for us. And we don't owe anyone an explanation as to why we've made them and, therefore, must let go of trying to justify them to everyone. We must also let go of the fear of being judged or misunderstood, and hope our loved ones are still able to find their way to support us, even if they don't fully understand our choices.

And the best way I know to do that is to talk and write, to share and live my truth authentically. Because when I live my life with such courage, the dementor of shame doesn't stand a chance, and I allow myself the space to accept, embrace and own my truth.

To truly let the world see me.

Practice Happy

"Do you *really* do all of this stuff yourself?"

A question of curiosity and bait and switch from two of my clients this week.

By "stuff" they meant the to-do list of self-care I have been recommending to them for a while now.

For the first time in probably my entire career, I was able to say, "Yes!"

Therapists struggle, too. We struggle with being brave. We have difficulty in some of our relationships. We make mistakes. We too can suffer from anxiety and depression. We have hurts and traumas. We have shame. And we fall off the wagon of good self-care, ultimately struggling to practice what we preach and teach.

In other words, we're human.

I didn't become a therapist for the money or the freedom of being self-employed, the money isn't that good for how difficult the job is and the freedom comes with a lot of sacrifices. I became a therapist because of back surgeries, a year in a body cast, depression, anxiety and the ultimate life didn't turn out how I wanted, failed infertility treatments. My story, my struggles, and flaws, all brought me to exactly where I needed to be, helping others. My story has always helped me to be a good therapist. However, the work I've done myself after enduring the losses of IVF has helped make me the best version of myself, and therefore an even better therapist.

Surviving IVF, but more importantly, choosing to thrive after the losses of IVF, has culminated into changing my entire life. I've changed the way I eat, the way I move, how I cope and how I take care of myself.

I chose to change.

Because when we experience trauma and loss, like that endured in the infertility journey, no matter what you get out of it, we can no longer go back to who you once were, even if we have no idea who that once was.

I chose the work of change to get back to the real me; me, who I honestly, hardly even remember ever existing.

This work has included everything I have always taught to my clients and more. But now, I practice it myself every day. I don't do it perfectly, and there are definitely the days I stand in my way and fall off track, to only then have to shake it off and begin again. I practice it daily so I can model to the people in my life, clients and loved ones, that it is possible and worth it. I practice it so I can push them forward and cheer them on. I practice it so I can empathize with how easy it is to get off track. And, I practice it because, without it, I'd still be in a ball at the bottom of a deep, dark cavern of my own grief and shame.

This practice is time-consuming and a downright pain in the ass some days. But I know if I make it a priority and indeed practice it all, my life will continue to improve. So every day I try to exercise, dance (stupid dance, really just bouncing around, spinning and kicking to my happy songs), meditate (even just 10 minutes of deep breathing helps), read, write, journal, color (yes in an actual coloring book with colored pencils and markers), do yoga (which is never very pretty), listen to happy music (my favorites are *Roar, Brave, Shake It Out, Rise, Rise Up* and anything played on JoyFM the St. Louis Christian station), play with my dogs, and watch something happy or funny or uplifting (www.24hoursofhappy.com or www.upworthy.com). There are days where everything on this list gets done, and then there are the days that life only allows enough time for a few. But I know, we all can make the time to do a good portion of this list every single day, whether or not it is cutting out 30 minutes of television or turning off the technology for an hour at night.

The best part? I promise it's worth it.

Practicing all this self-care provides me the strength and the space to live as my authentic self in this crazy world that often tells me I am not enough. With this, I live feeling the fear and being brave, embracing my flaws and losses, and living my authentic truth with all intensity and weirdness shining brightly.

So, I practice happy to *be* happy. And, I choose, every day, to live the true spirit of ever upward.

Embracing It to Truly Let It Go

"You have to go see *Frozen*!" my client texted me. "It is about everything you always talk about in our sessions: accepting ourselves and being vulnerable."

She also added that the music was amazing and Olaf the snowman was hysterical. So on that Tuesday after seeing several clients, I went and saw a children's movie in the middle of the afternoon…by myself. And I will fully admit, it was the perfect afternoon!

My client was right, the film was laugh out loud funny and the music was truthful, inspiring and captivating! All of this, and an amazing message that wasn't all about prince charming saving the girl. And, it totally backed up what I teach to my clients every day and how I try to live my own life; accept, let go and live your authentic truth. The title track, *Let It Go*, being the perfect vehicle to deliver all of these messages.

The theme of embracing who we are, accepting ourselves and moving through has also been the popular topic in my office this week. Every day I work with clients on their struggles; their anxieties or depression, their addictions or negative coping. I try to help them find the balance of learning the lesson in order to change and improve, while also accepting themselves. We all have our struggles, our fears, our weaknesses and faults. We all have our traumas, losses and flaws. Living our authentic truth means finding a way to make all of these things part of who we are and not all of our identity. Finding this balance myself has been the biggest challenge and change in me after IVF. It takes work to embrace and accept that I will never be a mother in the traditional sense, but embrace and accept I must do because that is the only way I will have the strength to let go of the yuck shit that comes with it all.

Before this wholehearted work, some used to call me angry. I would refute and say I was passionate. Looking back after the work I have done, and continue to do every day, I admit that more times than not my passion did come across as agitation, perhaps even anger. I completely inherit this characteristic from my dad; we have a lot of passion and if we are not careful it very easily becomes agitation and anger.

I feel it all, all at the same time and I feel it hard, And, I am an emoter on top of it, when I feel it, you see it!

What I have found is that if I am not mindful, it can be one of my major flaws and road blocks to happiness. However, I've also come to realize that it is not necessarily a part of my personality that I can "get rid of", but instead have to learn to manage better.

Surviving IVF and thriving after the major loss of motherhood dreams, I was forced to look at myself and truly change for the better. I had to redefine my happy. I will never not be fiery, it is everything of who I am. I feel every emotion, a lot. I see every side of everything, all of the time. I am intense, passionate…too much.

This is who I am. It is what I am learning to love about myself. But, it is also the part of me I must cope with to make it work *for* me. I must embrace the passion to let go of the distress.

I am passionate, and it is the single most important part of who I am, for it is what makes me the friend and the therapist I am. Fighting this part of me only crushes my authentic spirit. Being fearful of what others may think to the point of being defined by it only keeps me from accepting myself.

So maybe the key to letting it go is actually embracing it. Just as Elsa in *Frozen*, when we embrace the very fear that is holding us back it allows us to love and accept ourselves.

Only when we embrace our failings, our faults, our weaknesses, and our losses do they no longer become all of who we are. Through this embrace they become the things we can learn to manage, love and let go.

Making Room for the Light

We loathe discomfort. We can't stand to feel sad. Depression and anxiety make us want to escape our bodies. We all struggle to feel the unpleasantness of life. We struggle so much we often times go to any length to self-medicate and numb. Whether we drink or use. Or shop or gamble. Or watch hours of mind numbing television. Or pull our hair. Or binge and purge. We would so much rather hurt ourselves in the long term because all of these things provides us some sense of very temporary relief.

And, they work.

My clients are shocked when I say their "vices" (or in some cases addictions) are doing something positive for them. We, as human beings, don't do things that don't feel good or work. It's just many times these very things that work to numb us out to our pains and hurts often times stop working at some point, and they begin to create even more problems, especially shame and darkness.

I think, at times, emotions can become one of these vices, especially anger. Anger tends to be an emotion that many of us are comfortable feeling. Many of us would rather feel anger than sadness, as we kid ourselves into thinking it is easier. But, anger is a secondary emotion, behind it almost always fear, shame, loneliness or hurt. What I am learning about myself, after spending the last year of my life changing everything after the losses endured with IVF, is that this anger is definitely my go-to emotion. The bitter, and thank God very fleeting anger, the anger I've worked so hard on coping with and letting go of, but still seems to swoop in to save me. I hate this anger, especially because I want to let go of the biggest trigger for it.

I love children, I love when my loved ones get to have children; I even love when strangers, hell, people I don't even like get to have children. But where I am still struggling is with the people who "don't deserve" them. The super fertile 16 year olds. The couple who have already lost custody of their other 3 children. The people who don't even want them. I'm sure this list could go on and on, just watch the news.

And as usual, no emotion is uncomplicated for a therapist. This brief, but very strong, bitter angry emotion momentarily knocks me down. As I continue to do the work to redefine myself, I'm learning to rise strong out of it more quickly. I'm also understanding more about myself and how I feel about it.

Yes feeling about a feeling, oh the professional hazards of being a therapist!

– I am NO ONE to judge who gets the joy of children. I am neither judge nor jury, nor do I want to be.

– I do have faith that there are no mistakes, at least in the long run.

– Even though it feels really, really fucking unfair, it really is neither fair nor unfair, but it just is, and it is not mine to necessarily understand right now.

– And most importantly, I am coming to understand that this anger is coming in to save me from feeling what I really feel… which is simply really sad shame.

And that is okay. Sometimes things are just sad. It's sad IVF didn't work for us. It's sad we lost our 3 babies. It's sad we lost those 3 dreams. Giving myself permission to continue to feel that sadness, as needed, will help to stave off the anger that seems to set me back so much every time. I have to embrace it in order to let it go. When I allow myself to feel it, I don't become it. And only when I do this, is there enough space to truly find the ever upward. The ever upward that is this work of learning to be happy and healthy, and even okay and fulfilled, without children.

We all must work to accept that we are not wired to escape ourselves, no matter how hard we try. We have to feel, we have to feel it all, even the darkness, because when we allow ourselves to do that, it will pass and make room for the light.

The Frankenstein Walk

Making the impossible decision to stop IVF treatments, not adopt and figure out life childfree not by choice has been, at times, a daily Frankenstein walk.

That 'I have no idea how this works' walk.

That 'hold your arms out in front of you to break your fall' walk.

That 'really stiff legged how do these things work' walk.

That really, really ugly walk.

The 'I'm just figuring out how to do this' walk.

This walk includes fighting that feeling of never fitting in. I am quite literally always the only woman in her 30's without children everywhere I go. Rather, I must find my sense of belonging from within.

This walk includes owning my story and speaking it out loud for the world because it is only with speaking that I educate, but more importantly, honor myself and the work I have done.

This walk includes understanding my anger to really feel the most difficult emotion of grief in order to truly embrace and accept my childfree life.

This walk also still includes the ugly steps of figuring out what to do with the sense of feeling left behind.

My friends who are moms are some of my best and most supportive friends, especially on this journey. They are super women (even though, a lot of the time, they need to remind themselves that they don't necessarily need to be). They are the best women I know. All working full time, whether in or outside the home, and are the hardest working people I know. I admire their patience, their unconditional love and their unending strength. And there are simply no words for how amazing their love, support and understanding has been for me throughout this continued journey.

They are also, naturally, the busiest people on earth; raising children, nurturing a marriage and trying to find the time to sleep and do some basic self-care. They have practices 2 nights a week, games and birthday parties on the weekends and can book up their weekends with other families who have children pretty quickly.

And, sometimes there just isn't time for me, for us, the couple without kids.

And that's okay. And I do get it.

But, there are times I feel like I want to jump up and down, frantically waving my arms, screaming to them, "But I'm still here!"

I do still have a life I'd like to share with you.

I do still want to hear all about yours.

I do still need you to maintain our friendship.

Ending IVF and living a childfree life can very easily mean I lose my peer group. The crushing blow of not being able to fulfill my dream of motherhood means I have more time; more time for self-care, more time for my marriage, more time for my friendships. I suppose this can be an 'ever upward' of failed IVF and accepting a childfree life. However, it also can definitely feel pretty isolating, as most of my friends, especially my mom friends, don't necessarily have this 'luxury'.

So I am finding my Frankenstein walk, and figuring this all out along the way.

Working hard to maintain my friendships, even if at times it can feel like it is one sided. Because although some friendships may not survive the family with children versus childfree dynamic, most of mine do have the true grit (and importance to me) to make sure they do survive.

Building other friendships, perhaps finding other couples without children.

Making sure my mom friends know I'm here and that I treasure their friendships more than they will ever know.

But most importantly, learning to acknowledge and work on this sense of feeling left behind, because ultimately, I probably need to check myself.

Am I trying to fit in, when I need to trust that I always belong?

Am I holding on to anger, when I need to embrace sadness?

Am I honoring myself?

Am I putting enough effort into my friendships?

Am I being a friend to myself?
And, am I asking for what I want and need?
Because only when I am doing this work, will my
friends be walking alongside me, Frankenstein walk and all.

Our Fellow Warriors

We all have the basic needs for love and belonging, and we oftentimes believe that feeling understood goes hand in hand with this need.

However, it is impossible to be understood by everyone in our lives. This does not mean we aren't loved, but rather at times our loved ones just don't have it in them to really get it.

Or to really get us.

Surviving IVF and living a childfree life sometimes feels like I will never be fully understood.

For the most part, I have been lucky and blessed to have amazing people in my life. Even if they don't completely get the IVF thing, they work very hard on loving me through it. But, I have noticed a few categories have emerged:

My fellow warriors
Those who have been through some version of infertility or pregnancy loss themselves, even if their journey has looked completely different (especially their outcome).
They genuinely get it.
With them I am truly known.

My true friends (really family, chosen family).
Those who may have never had to think about infertility, never really been exposed to it and therefore struggle to empathize with the journey but they still try.
They ask the questions, sometimes not in the best way, but they still ask.
They truly walk along beside.
With them I am truly seen.

My limited supporters
Those who will never ask about it and become extremely uncomfortable whenever it's brought up.
They do their best with what they have.
With them I am truly loved.

My incapables.

Those who openly criticize, question and deny what I have been through. Maybe they used to talk and ask about it, but have never had the capacity to quite understand any of it. Not only do they deny the journey, but often times somehow shut down that part of who I am.

They will probably never get it.

With them I feel invisible.

This has nothing to do with my IVF journey at all, but rather is just what happens for all of us as we grow, evolve and love.

Relationships change, relationships end, relationships reemerge, relationships evolve.

As I hugged a dear friend good bye today, I am flooded with gratitude for change. The change of life, the change of relationships and how much we all change and grow. A friend who has been in and out of my life for years, some of our falling outs worse than others, but a friend who I know will always have some piece in my life and in my heart. We've had to re-categorize each other several times in our 17 year friendship.

I use the term re-categorize with my clients a lot, referring to the ever-changing relationships in our lives as we grow up. I believe people are meant to come in and out of our lives as we all change. Sometimes these changes warrant a re-categorization. Who you thought would always be there may leave your life for a few years and then reemerge. Or they may be gone forever, never meant to be the lifelong friend you had hoped. It is true that some people are simply meant for a season.

Hand in hand with re-categorization, we all must accept the limitations of our loved ones. Sometimes, they just don't have what we need. Accepting their limitations improves our well-being, as we only have control over ourselves. We cannot *make* someone understand us. Accepting our loved ones' limitations means we realize they just don't have it to give. We must stop going to the empty well looking for water.

Being completely understood by others needs to have nothing to do with who we are or our stories. We must honor ourselves, no matter what our loved ones' capabilities of understanding us are.

We all must do the work to validate ourselves; seeing, knowing and loving ourselves.

Life is difficult and people are complicated, which means relationships take work and are forever changing.

For me, I must accept that there are some who will *never* understand my journey of infertility or the lifelong losses of a childfree life. And even though this can feel like a complete denial of who I am and may change our relationship, I must continue to speak my truth and live my story authentically for the world to see, because this is simply who I am.

With this acceptance, I will however never stop going to the well. Because I believe people can change and grow. I am a therapist for God's sake. Every single day I work with clients on changing themselves and therefore their lives. But, I will go to the well for the sunshine and flowers, doing the work to never expect water to be in that empty well.

I must live my truth, not to fulfill the need to feel understood or to make someone get it, but rather to live my authentic truth and light.

To be true to myself.

For that light will reveal my fellow warriors and true friends.

And maybe, one day, that light will grow those limited supporters and incapables into my ever upwards.

And, perhaps help shine someone out of their darkness.

Wallow

I will fully admit I have rough days, as we all do.
But the other day I wallowed.
I *really* wallowed for a bit.
Going to the OB/GYN is never fun for a woman, but it can definitely be hell for a childless not by choice woman; let alone getting news that it is quite possible that IVF triggered my useless ovaries to develop painful cysts which are now causing major back pain. On top of seemingly always having to remind the nurse that IVF didn't work for us, there is no baby, and yes we are done trying.
This day, I cried.
I pouted.
I talked.
"I'm frustrated."
"I'm pissed".
"It's not fucking fair."
Then life somehow pulls you out if it, but only if you have your eyes wide open to it.
I had some amazing sessions with clients. I reminded myself of my own session with my therapist. The puppies finally played in the deep snow and made me laugh just when I needed to. And three of my favorite little boys left me a voicemail and sent me a video text message.
As my therapist reminded me earlier that week, "You have chosen what to do with all of this. You could never *not* be *Ever Upward*; always growing, learning, changing, educating, evolving and figuring it out. "
And she's right
I didn't get to choose that I would spend a year of my life in a body cast after two back surgeries. I didn't get to choose that IVF did not work for us. And I definitely didn't choose that my body feels like it is rebelling against my childless status right now.
But I can choose resiliency. I can choose to speak the truth about IVF and loss. I can choose to connect with others through our stories. I can choose where I go from here and who I want to be. I can choose my ever upward.

My clients also reminded me that week as they continue to fight, change for the better and not be their pasts, their struggles, traumas or losses.

I choose to fight too.

My dogs reminded me to get out of my head and to just laugh; watching them play in the snow is pure joy.

I choose joy.

And finally, three of my favorite kiddos, begging me to come play Just Dance 2014... well nothing makes me smile more than that.

I choose love (and fun).

God, the Universe, whatever you call it, for me it is God, will always send us the exact message we need to remind us that there is a higher purpose to our journey.

We simply have to be open enough to receive it and then choose it.

So wallow, but just for a bit, we are totally allowed.

But be careful of sitting in the shit for too long, you just might miss the message; the moment of pure joy, the love, the choice of your ever upward.

Taking Off the Armor of My Choice

Publishing a book and blog for the entire world to read, means one must be ready for the critics, even the really unforgiving, judgmental and unsympathetic ones.

Sometimes they are strangers on the other side of the world and other times they are your very own loved ones.

I've experienced my first super harsh critic. And one who said the words I have feared the greatest, *You CHOSE to not have kids.*

Publicly starting the conversation that it is okay to stop IVF treatments before getting the intended, desired, wished for, hoped for, prayed for, and yes, even paid for result of a baby is not the most mainstream message, let alone publicly owning our decision to not adopt. These continue to be some of the scariest things I write and speak about.

Scary because I have ultimately feared this exact judgment.

What if people think I did not want kids bad enough because we didn't do 5 or 10 years of treatments? What if people think I did not want kids bad enough because I'm willing to admit that adoption isn't right for us?

What if people think I didn't want to be a mom enough?

Which boils down to the usual shitty first draft, as we say in the Rising Strong™ work of Brené Brown, I am not enough.

Maybe to some, I have chosen to not be a mother.

But I know my truth.

I fought really hard to be a mother. I paid lots of money to be a mother. I endured painful tests and procedures to be a mother. I put my body through synthetic hormonal hell to be a mother. I put my faith and trust into many doctors and other humans to be a mother.

Does accepting that the battle would never have my desired outcome mean I chose to not be a mom? Does redefining my life and figuring out childfree mean I chose to not be a mom? Does accepting what is mean I chose to not be a mom?

Maybe to some, this is my choice to not have children. But, I know I tried to be a mom, in fact, I know I am a mom.

And, though, I respect your opinion I will not be defined by it.

I am working every day to accept graciously that I will never be a mom in the traditional sense.

And I know, accepting this as my truth doesn't mean I didn't want it.

And I know, redefining everything doesn't mean I chose not to have kids.

I have chosen what I can. I have accepted what is.

And I write about it, to help and heal myself, and hopefully others.

And I will not apologize for that, as I choose to be my own witness in search of others; my warriors and friends.

And the only thing scarier than publicly owning all of this as my truth?

Would be not owning it.

Sometimes we don't get what we want or what we dreamed of or what we fought really hard for, what we feel is meant as ours, or even, what we paid for.

Does anyone really?

Sometimes we lose our way, our truth, our dreams and faith.

But, sometimes it is through these very never meant to be's that we find ourselves, our journey and our truth.

No matter the judgments and shaming and misunderstanding, this is my story of not just proving it, but owning it.

So be clear as I clarify for my critics, I will not armor up, I will not shy away and I will not stop living my authentic truth.

Because this is my ever upward.

Lights in a Tunnel

I can't keep doing this.
Things will never get better.
Why can't I just do this?
I've never been able to change before.
It will never work.
Will I ever get better?
It's too hard.
Why can't I stop?
It's too good to be true.
It won't last.
Why do I keep doing this?
I can't.
I won't.

The words of battle scars. The words of recovery wars lost thus far. The words of pain, hurt, loss and shame.

The words before the true fight.

Life is hard, people are complicated and we simply just don't get the joy without the pain and work. Which means it can be tempting to give up, to quit; to accept what is but not in the healthy-letting-go-way and only in the learned-helplessness-give-up way.

Sometimes we can't even fathom putting one foot in front of the other because we're still trying to pull ourselves back up from falling.

Sometimes we simply cannot see the light at the end of the tunnel anymore.

Dark hopelessness.

Except, I can always see your light.

~

I help.

I can't not help.

And, I love what I do. I was born to do what I do. My life, and my survivals, have made me very good at what I do. Every day I fight alongside amazing people who are setting forth to change their own lives. To choose themselves. To choose to fight. To choose their ever upward.

This war of change can, at times, feel like the most impossible choice ever. But it is also the most necessary choice ever. And it is a war that is won through each small battle, each small step taken forward in that long dark tunnel of recovery. That tunnel that, hopefully, you can see the light at the end of.

But oftentimes, this just isn't how it works. We will want to quit and the light will disappear and we will even lose some of the battles. But that is exactly when I ask my clients to have faith. Because, when they can no longer see their light at the end of the tunnel I need them to trust that I can see it for them.

Because that light just isn't their recovery, it is their light, the light of their spirit, soul, being.

I need them to trust that I can see who they are truly meant to be

That I can see what really lies beneath all of the struggle.

I see them, I see their light. Always.

~~~

But, sometimes that light isn't always at the end of the tunnel. Sometimes, in our fight to get back to our true selves the tunnel can work against us, creating a blind tunnel vision. The tunnel vision that keeps us stuck. That keeps us trying the same things over and over that just aren't working. We have been losing the battles and have to force ourselves to put one foot in front of the other with our heads down because we simply don't have the strength in us to keep going if we look up and see that the light isn't there anymore.

But this is when we miss it. This dark stuckness that keeps our heads down makes us completely miss the lights beside us. The other outs. The other helps. The hands reaching out for us.

The lighted detours.

I work every day to not only see the lights within my clients, but to also remind them of that light throughout their journey through the dark tunnels of recovery. But it is also my job to help them find the other lights beside them; these lighted detours.

Because recovery isn't this straight up trajectory of perfection. It is usually hell filled with deep dry valleys, cold thin aired mountains, swamps, quicksand pits and even tight ropes across ravines. And it has many detours, both darkened and blinding detours.

Recovery definitely includes those darker detours, the ones that just didn't work. We didn't quite make the best choice possible. And a lot of the times, this can set us back, but never back to the beginning and we just need to take the best next step. It is then that we must remember to keep our eyes open to those lighted detours. The detours that we easily miss because we are trudging along so painstakingly in the war of recovery searching for the light at the end of the tunnel.

Many times, these lighted detours can be our outs. Our escape from the cycle of hurt. The path to our recovery. Our lighted path to our ever upward.

Recovery, from whatever, is brutal, the tunnel is almost always long and dark. Having someone to walk alongside you through that path is helpful beyond measure. Someone who can always see your light. Someone who can see the light at the end for you when you lose track. Someone who can remind you of your own light. Someone to nudge you to look over to the lighted detours.

Someone to fight for you, but most importantly, with and alongside you.

We Hold the Pieces to Our Puzzle

Every day I work with clients to help them learn how to let go, accept, redefine and find themselves. Often times we work on owning our stories and not allowing our whole selves to be defined by something that has happened to us, a mistake we've made or a loss or trauma we have suffered. A lot of what I do is help my clients figure out how to be happy and healthy after things do not end up how they had hoped for, pictured or planned for. I help, I teach and I model, as I have fought this recovery battle myself.

We all have an epic story, and we all have hardship in our lives. Because hard is hard. Where we often get tripped up is in how we integrate these pieces of our stories into our whole, and hopefully one day, thriving selves.

I often get asked things like...

"How long will I hold onto this?"

"Will this ever get easier?"

"Will I ever stop thinking about it?"

Here's the thing, our lives are our puzzles.

Our life, our story, is a million piece jigsaw puzzle made up of pieces in every color, size and shape possible.

A puzzle that will always have some missing pieces.

As it takes our lifetime to complete it.

A puzzle that will have missing pieces forever, if we don't face the work we need to do to recover from whatever we need to recover from; leaving an incomplete picture if we don't do this work. Sure, we may not notice the gaping holes in the whole picture from afar, but when we really look closely they will be impossible to ignore.

As they are missing pieces of us.

A puzzle that only we hold all the pieces to.

When we do the work that we need to live a happy, fulfilled, authentically brave life and to heal ourselves we place every puzzle piece into place. We not only place each piece into it's perfect home, we also push it down.

Therefore, making the seamless picture of our intricately flawed, and yet perfectly imperfect beautiful lives.

Sure up close, one will see all the individual pieces of our stories but from afar they will simply see us.

All of us.

We are made up of all the pieces of our puzzle; each moment of our lives completing the picture and each story defining parts of who we are.

But, we must remember we hold the pieces ourselves, as we have the power for change and recovery.

We have the power to complete our puzzle and therefore truly, and bravely, embrace and own all the pieces of us.

My First Step Out of Rock Bottom

We had already made the impossible decision of stopping IVF treatments without having become parents and knew that adoption was not for us.

Surely, this was it, the worst it could get.

I had already survived two back surgeries, one year in a body cast, depression, two rounds of failed IVF with a gestational surrogate, three lost babies, depression again, anxiety, and anger.

But that is the important part, I had only survived up until that point. And then I was pushed to the edge of doubt and question, the edge of even worse; we had to the make the even more impossible decision to let go of our first furry child, Maddie.

Maddie, my little yorkie poo, who I got when I was single and living in the big city. Maddie, who took to love Chad more than me when he came into my life. Maddie, who was the weirdest, least trained and biggest pain in the ass dog ever.

Maddie, our first child was dying.

And there I found myself, off that edge right in my rock bottom.

Dark.

Pain.

Nothing.

Anger.

I can't say for sure what was the one catalyst for me to take the first giant, and most difficult, step out of rock bottom. That first step of my own walk on the moon. The first step that has been my life in recovery ever since.

I know it was a combination of finding the work of Brené Brown and learning how to own all the parts of my story with bravery in order to live my now wholehearted life.

I know it was the decision to change my lifestyle by changing my food and exercise and getting off medication and starting yoga, meditation, self-compassion and beginning the tough wrestle of my faith.

Above all, I know it was a decision, my choice.

My choice to no longer be the victim to my past, to my traumas, to my losses. To no longer just survive and choose to thrive.

My daily, sometimes minute-by-minute choice, to choose to thrive these survivals. To place these amazing and haunting hurts into my life puzzle making them the beautiful tapestry of my life thus far, and therefore just part of my epic story.

My every step on my moon. My walk that continues with many lights of my own ever upward.

Starting to write.

Owning my story and publishing the blog and first book.

Improving my relationships, including setting boundaries.

Finding, creating, asking for and receiving my child*full* life.

Investing in my career, and therefore myself.

Re-awakening my marriage after the traumas and losses of IVF.

Fighting for my faith and finally finding a church where I belong with Him.

To wake up and stand up.

To consider it *all* pure joy.

My walk on the moon started at my rock bottom with a damn near impossible, but completely necessary choice.

The choice, my choice, of the first step of my walk, for myself, my recovery, my happiness, my ever upward.

My Dementor

For a while I gave presentations as a Lunch and Learn at a major corporation in St. Louis. Before my sixth learning lunch with this company, I had a shame meltdown, which feels ridiculous, especially because I always have good attendance, great feedback and they actually pay me pretty well to speak.

And yet that morning I over-prepared and I literally made myself sick with anxiety and self-doubt.

Because, that day I spoke on Wholehearted Parenting.

And, I am not a parent.

And, I was scared shitless.

A few days before the presentation my shame consumed me, "I am not a parent and I am speaking on parenting and this is complete public knowledge now".

The self-doubt settled over me like a thick fog casting fear inside my very core.

Shame.

Fucking shame.

Like the dementor to my light, stealing my voice, sucking away my soul, leaving my heart empty.

I reached out to my friend, Janine, who organizes the talks and she of course gave me an amazing pep talk. And then the night before my friend and colleague reminded me that I am actually a parent. Kelly's words will forever and always mean the world to me. She said that I parent as much as she does as a mother to two boys, just in different ways; I parent my dogs and I parent all of the children in my life and that most of all I parent my clients. In many ways therapy is like parenting or even re-parenting with clients. She parents her two boys, but my audience of children is simply bigger as this is my purpose, and my path.

I cried and took in her words because I knew they were my truth. I drew in a deep knowing breath and thanked her for reminding me of my light. She reminded me of what I know every day in many ways, I wasn't given the chance or blessing of my own children because I am meant for this greatness of working with clients, writing and helping others. It's neither better nor worse or more or less important, it's just different.

So, that morning before I walked into that board room I wrote myself a permission slip, just like we ask ourselves and clients to do as they work through The Daring Way™ and Rising Strong™ curriculum. I wrote myself my permission slip and set it right beside my notes.

I have permission to be scared. I have permission to not be parent enough. I have permission to know, and own, that I know what I am talking about and that I can help even though I am not a parent in the traditional sense.

And so I spoke. I was painfully vulnerable in owning to them that I am not a parent but that I was there to teach them about wholehearted parenting. I called out my own imposter syndrome, and let them in to my world: I don't get to be a parent but I can still help you be a better one I think.

I also stated that I am the right person to do that because, one, I actually have the time to read the research and parenting books because I wasn't able to be a mom. And two, I parent every single day, just not my own children (and according to Kelly this probably means my house is cleaner, I am more well rested and I have more sex).

I was real, I was vulnerable and I allowed my brilliant light to outshine my shame. And because I fought for that bravery, I connected and delivered one of my best lectures. I left that presentation having no doubt that there would be some families that weekend with some new language and new ways to love and parent because of that hour we spent together.

Doing the work of recovery and learning shame resilience doesn't mean we won't experience shame. It simply means that we will be able to better cope with it when it does come in.

Shame is my dementor. And it can be very ominous, floating over me threatening to take my spirit. So, I must choose to rise, live with courage and rewrite my story.

Chosen Children

A picture mail text of Lyla's drawing of us.
Snail mail of Joycelyn's drawing of the dogs.
A picture mail text of Lane with his "Justine socks" on.
A voice mail from the boys begging us to come play Just Dance.
My favorite picture of the boys cuddling with the three dogs watching cartoons.
A birthday card from McKinley.
The moms in my life will never know how much the small gestures of letting me know their children are thinking of me mean to me; as they mean the world.
I will forever spend my energy making sure these children know I love them and I am here for them and more than anything I want, and really need, to be part of their lives.
As, these are our chosen children.
The children we have the honor of being godparents to. The children we have the privilege of being their guardians. The children we get to see grow up. The children who ask to see us. The children who love us. The children we love more.
Or maybe, it's really that they are the children who have chosen us.
Surviving the losses of IVF and accepting a childfree life to redefine family for us has meant we figure out what it means to still have children in our lives. It means living my truth as a woman who wanted, and desperately, tried to have her own children. It means having the courage to say adoption isn't for us. And yet, it is also making sure my heart is not closed off to all the light and love that family and children can bring to my life, even if it comes with the bittersweet sadness that they aren't my own.
It means traveling to Vegas for McKinley's birthdays.
It means going to Noah's piano recitals.
It means sending happy birthday and happy valentine's videos of the dogs singing to all of the kids.
It means having a toy room in my house.
It means having the pool for everyone to enjoy all summer long.
It means watching the boys play the Wii for hours.

It means embracing my sadness that I will never get to parent in the traditional sense, in order to make room for the endless, ever upward light that all of these families and kids bring to my life every single day.

Because it would be even more sad to cut children out of my life completely because it hurt too badly. To not honor the mother I am, the mother I fought so hard to become, and not have the glory of children in my life would only make the sad even sadder. That alternative is too dark. So I choose to love on them, to let them love me and to honor the mom I am.

I do it because it is my journey. I do it because I have fought for my recovery. I do it because it is ever upward.

And, because we have all chosen each other.

The Childfree Mother

I am not a mother.

I wanted to be a mother.

I fought very hard to be a mother.

I paid a lot of money and put my body (and my surrogate's body) through synthetic hormonal hell to be a mother.

But, I am not a mother.

At least in the common definition of mother.

And yet, here I am, a fan of Glennon Melton, her *Momastery* blog and her book *Carry On, Warrior*, contributing to her Messy, Beautiful Warrior Project... but I am not a mother.

Talk about messy and scared to death.

But I choose beautiful and courage instead.

My story could be considered epically sad and tremendously messy. But, I like to think of it as beautifully flawed and filled with ever upward light and love, and every piece of my life puzzle in this Messy, Beautiful life is proof that I am a Warrior. Because, it is messy and beautiful to live our lives authentically brave, and so, every single day I choose to live as a Messy, Beautiful Warrior.

Being a warrior means living all the parts of my story fully, wholeheartedly and brazenly authentically courageous.

It means never shying away from the most asked question of every woman my age, "How many children do you have?", and answering it in my own honest way.

"We tried, we tried really hard, but we can't have kids."

It means never allowing shame to steal my story when I am asked the inevitable second most asked question, "Well, why don't you just adopt?"

"We know adoption is not our path. We've been through a lot, financially and emotionally, with In Vitro Fertilization (IVF), surrogacy and losing three babies already. We have decided to accept a childfree not by choice life."

I will not apologize if my answer makes you uncomfortable. I will not allow your need to fix or take away my pain to silence my story. I will not let shame, self- or societal-induced, steal my light.

So I will educate. I will write and speak my story, owning my shame, every day of my life. I will live it because it is the only way to honor myself. I will live it because it is the only way the landscape of infertility will change. I will live it because we all have our epically Messy, Beautiful journeys. Because hard is hard and maybe, just maybe, openly owning my story will make you just uncomfortable enough to open your eyes and heart to someone else's story and therefore lead you to some compassion and understanding.

In short, my life and the stories I write in *Ever Upward* are the epitome of Messy, Beautiful. They are about what happens when we don't get what we so desperately wanted and hoped for. What happens when we don't get what we thought we deserved?

Ever Upward is about letting go of what isn't and embracing a new purpose.

Every day I live and write about my Messy, Beautiful.

Every day I live and write about the epic stumbles followed by every purposeful rise.

My messy is the random anger and bitterness that can over take me at times. My messy is the underlying sadness that comes and goes because I didn't get what I wanted or hoped for. My messy is that in every traditional sense of a woman my age, I won't ever really fit in because I am not a mother. My messy is owning my struggle in my recovery.

But, I choose beautiful in my ever upward mess.

My beautiful is surviving failed IVF and surrogacy. My beautiful is accepting and redefining my childfree life. My beautiful is finding my chosen family within the love of our surrogate family especially with their unexpected pregnancy after our failed IVF tries. My beautiful is finding my role in the lives of all our chosen children. My beautiful is having the patience to find my faith again. My beautiful is owning my story, for the world to see, in order to break the silence of infertility but more importantly in claiming my ongoing recovery. My beautiful is knowing that I am a mother in more ways than most are open to considering. My beautiful is in trusting my gut wrenching ironic path to my ever upward light in being a childfree mother.

As, my beautiful is living my light, authentically brave, mess and all, no matter what. Because life in recovery is always a messy, beautiful ever upward journey.

Mourning What Should Have Been

significant part of me cringes as I put the word *should* in the title of this essay. As a therapist who works a lot with helping people change their thinking I have attempted to erase should from my vocabulary. I also work with my clients to do the same. As some therapists say, "Don't should all over yourself!" Should is typically riddled with guilt and shame and just yuck. What do we need and want? Not, what should we... Change should to need or want and feel the difference, both when you speak to yourself and when expecting things from your loved ones.

I should go to the gym.
Do I need or want to go to the gym? Or as Louise Hay recommends, If I really wanted to go to the gym, could i?
He/She should know how I'm feeling right now.
I need to tell him/her how I feel and what I want.
I shouldn't feel sad any longer.
Do I need or want to figure out this sadness still or is it time to release it?

~~~~

I wrote my first post for *Ever Upward* five short months ago. Never could I have dreamed how much my life would change. Never could I have dreamed how many amazing people I would "meet". Never could I have dreamed how much our stories are all connected and the embrace I've felt through this connection.

This connection has only been further solidified through my participation in Momastery's Messy, Beautiful Warrior Project. Our stories, all messy and all beautiful, are what connect us to one another. I think, our stories, even more so, are what connect us back to ourselves. And, it seems our stories tend to have the major theme I oftentimes see with my clients every day: mourning what should have been or what we thought should have been.

I think at times, at least for me, it can feel like these should have beens determine my everything; my every day, and even my every minute. And if I don't practice the work of my recovery, I risk the should have beens taking over and defining my entire being. Just Google something like *letting go of what isn't* and you will be overwhelmed by thousands of quotes on how we must let go of what isn't in order to make room for what can be. In reality, this has probably been the major encompassing theme of *Ever Upward* from the beginning.

But what is striking me the most lately, is how much we judge others or lack empathy for others in regards to their mourning of their should have beens; their losses, their stories.

The very stories that seem and feel so different than ours, but I am realizing are so very much the same.

We all have should have beens...

I should have gone to school sooner.

I shouldn't have stayed so long.

I should have enjoyed my younger years more.

I should be able to forgive this by now.

I should have taken better care of my body.

I should have been more honest.

They shouldn't have left me.

I should be better by now.

I should have left them.

I should be over this.

This list could go on and on. Ultimately, aren't we all just trying to figure out how to let go of what didn't turn out? To redefine after all our shoulds didn't come true?

And of course, there are the should have beens of motherhood and family, especially considering these are the ones that seem to go unspoken and judged a lot.

Your child was born premature, you didn't get to hold him/her for weeks or months and you didn't get that happy bring them home day or first few months.

You were miserably sick your entire pregnancy and you honestly hated every second of it, while also being so thankful for it and therefore felt guilty.

You lost a child way too early for anyone to bear, let alone understand the lifelong losses that come with that grief.

You were never able to even hold that child or only held that child for a few heartbreaking but amazing hours.

You only achieved pregnancy through infertility measures and will never get to have wild drunk sex that ends up in your blessing of a child 40 weeks later.

You feel sad and guilty and mad that you didn't start trying sooner.

You weren't planning on getting pregnant and therefore spent most of it scared to death rather than relishing every second of it.

You are a birth mom.

You are a mom.

You adopted your child or children or embryos and are so thankful for children but grieve that you will never get to see you and your partner's genes combined.

You will never get to experience pregnancy yourself.

You have had to make major IVF decisions such as how many embryos to transfer, what to do with leftover embryos, what happens if you can't afford another round of treatments, etc., etc.

You are blessed with one or two or even three children but always wanted a big family and it doesn't seem to be happening, you feel the gamut of sadness, anger and guilt coupled with how lucky and blessed you are to have any children.

You are a stay at home mom but wish you were working.

You are a working mom but wish you were a stay at home mom.

You have happy and healthy children but your friends don't, and you feel blessed and lucky but guilty, especially when sometimes you'd really like Sunday completely to yourself, on the couch watching *The Walking Dead* all day long.

Your infertility is due to one partner or maybe the combination of you together and it creates frustration, sadness, guilt and maybe even blame.

I am sure I am missing many, many more here.

And then there is my story, I wanted to a mom, I tried to a mom but it is not my journey to have. And I've worked to accept a childfree life and fight for my recovery. But now for the first time, I am beginning to experience those feelings of relief, calm and even gratitude when my chosen children don't come home with us or they go to their own homes after visiting. Or that our Sunday is filled with whatever we want, even that day long marathon of The Walking Dead. Or that I don't have to negotiate over meal time or figure out how to attend 3 soccer games at once.

Does that mean I didn't want our three babies enough? Does that mean I'm not sad anymore? Or does that simply mean I'm figuring out how to let go of what I wanted and hoped for. That I am figuring out my mourning for what should have been, and learning to accept my true childfree life.

It's all so complicated; neither story better or worse or more difficult than the other. It's just life, which includes suffering for us all. And it is our sufferings and our recoveries from them that make us who we are. As David Brooks wrote for the New York Times in his article titled *What Suffering Does*, "Recovering from suffering is not like recovering from a disease. Many people don't come out healed; they come out different."

But it is through this ongoing process of healing, of figuring out what comes after the should have been, that we find ourselves and our story again.

Because, who are we to have the power to say what should have been?

I am not meant to be a mother, at least in the way I hoped, dreamed, planned and paid for.

Should I have been?

Perhaps. But, continuing to insist on the should only denies my truth.

But more importantly, who are we to judge or question one's grief around these sufferings or losses? Who are we to judge one for how they mourn their should have beens? Who are we to dare ask, "When are you going to get over it?"

We must figure out how we can give ourselves, and others, permission to mourn their should have beens? Can we give ourselves, and others, permission to feel it all; the blessings, the lucky, the anger, the sadness, the guilt, and even, the shame. And, to feel it all at the same time.

Because, really it is through these permissions that our recoveries can begin. It is within these permissions that I finally put the puzzle pieces into my bigger life story. It is within these permissions that I can allow myself the relief, and even gratitude, of a childfree life while also, at the very same time, feeling my sadness, anger and envy of your life with children.

It is within these permissions that we open up the space and light for the mourning of what should have been to become what needs to be.

The Authentic Therapist

"You see a therapist?!?"

I think this question is posed for several reasons. But, if I practiced mind reading, which I never recommend doing, this is what I think is really behind this question:

Only really crazy people have to see a therapist!

But you're a therapist, shouldn't you have this all figured out?

Chin up! Can't you just figure it out for yourself?

You must not be strong enough to deal.

~~~~

I struggle and I am a therapist.

I am a therapist, and yet I am also a perfectly imperfect human myself.

I have faith there will be a day when we all have a therapist we work with sporadically throughout our lives. Because life is hard and people are complicated. And to have someone outside of your friends and family to help you through it all, is nothing less than priceless.

I also have faith there will be a day that people aren't shocked that I regularly see a therapist (patients, friends, family and strangers alike). Because life is hard and people are complicated, especially when you are the one helping others through all that life is hard and people are complicated stuff.

I am also a therapist who lives my life afraid and brave every second of every day. I live my life honoring my authentic truth. I live this way because it is how I have found my own recovery. I live this way because I have done the hard work, choosing it every day, of my recovery. I live this way because I simply cannot not live this way.

I also live this way because I see how much my clients are empowered to change their own lives as I show them my work.

It was drilled into my head in graduate school that as counselor we DO NOT GIVE ADVICE! It didn't take long of me working in this field, in the real world of limited time and resources, managed health care and difficult life circumstances, that I knew this philosophy just wasn't going to work for the people I help or for me and the kind of therapist I wanted to be.

I will not answer all your troubles, I will not do the work for you, and I cannot save you if you are not ready to save yourself. But I can assure you, I will walk alongside you modeling what it is like to fight for your own recovery. I will pull you forward, at times, urging you to have faith that it will get better. And, there will be those times I push you forward because it is simply what you need right then to take the best next stop forward.

I also learned in graduate school, as is the philosophy of many in my field, that our clients know nothing about us, that we are blank slates. Early in my career, before I really had to fight for my own recovery, I practiced more on this side of impersonal connection. However, I found that I was working way harder than my clients. I also found I struggled with boundaries because I was fighting so much harder than the client to save their own life. Only after fighting for my own recovery was I able to both share and model my fight for my clients. Self-disclosure will always be a hotly debated topic in mental health, as it needs be. It needs to be used only when it will move the client forward in their own work. Therapists, myself included, must be careful to not dump our own shit onto our clients. Constantly keep tabs on why we are sharing our own battles with our clients to make sure it is for them and not us.

My own transparency along with the public forum of writing a memoir and blog has meant my clients may know a lot about my life and struggles, sometimes even before their first session. I am sure this will make some in my field cringe, graduate professors included. However, it is without a doubt, that I can say this has done nothing but make me a better therapist and better able to help others through their own struggles. Not only does this provide constant teaching moments for clients in empathy and authenticity but they know they are truly seen and known when they come to see me for their sessions. They know they are talking to someone who has fought this epic war of recovery. They know they are talking to someone who is not perfect, who also struggles with self-compassion towards that perfection but who, most importantly, owns their story. I have been asked by my own treatment team what it has been like for my clients to know more about my life, especially as this is something I make sure to have supervision on. Honestly, it is something that is difficult to put into words as it feels like something bigger than us; it is recovery, it is connection, it is ever upward.

Marianne Williamson captures this perfectly, "As we let our own light shine, we unconsciously give other people permission to do the same. As we are liberated from our own fear, our presence automatically liberates others."

So I will write about my life, both in my blog and in my books. I will share with my clients parts of my own story when I think it will be helpful in their recovery. I will model the daily fight and choices of recovery.

I will help.

I will walk alongside.

I will pull forward.

And, I will push.

I will help by being me. I will help by owning my story; ugly, shameful, scary, imperfect parts and all. Because it is only within this ownership that my ever upward is found and I can really help.

Almost Enough Moments

It is not uncommon for me to have a regular existential crisis, sometimes they even feel on schedule every couple of months. Between publishing *Ever Upward*, continuing to blog, fighting every day to share and spread the healthy messages in the infertility and loss community and work the jobs that pay the bills, and all while living my life in a wholehearted and brave way, this journey is not for the faint of heart. I often find myself feeling all sides of everything, over-feeling and over-thinking, doubting and just plain struggling.

How can I balance this desire for the blog to blow up and the book to get published, both for validation of my story and for the wider outreach to help others but also because I think it just has to with knowing my story has already touched and helped so many? How do I let go and trust that what is meant to happen will happen, as it has never been in my hands to begin with?

How do we sit with the be all, end all questions, what is this all supposed to mean? Why did this happen?

Aren't we all wondering the why?

Why does the 35 year old mother of two young children get late stage colorectal cancer?

Why did he cheat?

Why did she have to die?

Why did he have to fall?

Why did they leave?

Why didn't I die?

Why are they lying?

Why did this have to happen???

Why?

But, I'm not sure we will ever get to know the why.

And, what I think I am learning is that some of our answers can maybe be found in our almost enough moments.

You know those moments where you look up (to who or whatever you believe in, for me it is God) and say okay, *I get it*. I would not have this if that had all worked out. Or I would not have this if I had not lost that. But really, that just doesn't feel like it's quite enough? So we question it; *I get it, I am thankful, but it's still not enough for all that pain, all that suffering, the never to be's. I hope you have more and better in the works!*

I am also learning we all have to figure out how to open ourselves up to these almost enough moments, really embracing their potential for awe.

Can I have the presence and gratitude to embrace that piece of almost enough *and* have the faith that I might get to see the pieces all fit together one day? Better yet, can I have the presence and gratitude, and patience, enough to have the faith that I just may not get to see them all fit together and that the almost enough is, well, enough?

Because without a doubt, I have some pretty amazing almost enough moments...

- Being McKinley's godparents.
- Being asked to be in the delivery room to help bring Abigail Justine into this world.
- Having every moment with our chosen family.
- Attending all the piano recitals, church concerts and ball games of all our chosen children.
- My friends through Emerging Women, The Daring Way™ certification, my coaching communities and the blog.
- Our Christmas morning tradition of going to see what Santa brought our chosen children.
- The healing journey of writing my book.
- A better marriage.
- Building our family home, Mason house, for all our friends and family to grow and enjoy with us.
- The continuing journey of my blog.
- Becoming a better therapist.
- Our dogs.
- My improved relationships.
- The happier, healthier me.
- *Fighting for me, fighting for my recovery and rediscovering my light.*

I could go on and on, because I am able to wholeheartedly say, the list of my almost enough moments truly is endless.

My soul will always have the scars of my three lost babies, of three lost dreams, of three never to be's. But, I can choose if this is my whole story and I can also choose to move forward, having the faith that everything is exactly as it is supposed to be, no matter the why.

But, can I trust and have the patience that these almost enough moments will lead me to more understanding and that my suffering, better yet, my story, will end exactly as it is meant to? It is daily learning to have the patience and faith that I just might never get that final moment of what I think would be completion, understanding and the good enough reason for my sufferings.

So I must figure out how to be okay with that. I must learn to be whole without those enough moments. Trusting that the sole, better yet, soul, purpose I think I have found is really only my plan, and I'm not sure I really get that say.

But I also have to keep that in check with this part of me that yearns for my losses to mean something bigger; to change the world and help others. It is this part that asks, why else would I have been given this path in life? Why else would I have suffered the way I have and lost what I have? What would be the point of that? Am I that undeserving? Or is this my punishment for something? Surely, it has to mean something; two back surgeries, a year in a body cast, failed IVF with a surrogate, three lost babies and fighting for recovery can't just be it, can it?

And, there it is again… Why did this have to happen to me?

I am not sure these questions come from the best part of me. However, I also know I wouldn't be honoring myself if I didn't allow this doubt of mine a space to question; and maybe that is the point exactly.

There is only so much we are capable of, and probably allowed to, understand in this life. Maybe, it will always be this constant balance between finding my purpose through my story of struggle, making sure it means something more, at least to me, and trusting that it will still mean just as much without the soul completing clarity I so desire.

Because, all those almost enough moments…well, maybe it's up to me to embrace them as my ever upward, which really makes them the *more than enough moments*.

But, it has only been through my sufferings and my fight for recovery that I have been able to really see, let alone embrace, these moments as being more than enough.

My recovery.

My story.

My purpose.

My path.

My light.

And even, my soul scars.

Allowing every single almost enough moment to really be more than enough.

My True Witness of 30 Years

We've known each other since we were four years old.

She can tell you every single memory of our lives; what we were wearing, who was there, what was said and the craziness that ensued.

She probably knows me the best, as she has known me the longest. But, in reality, she probably knows me the best because she has witnessed my deepest lows and stood by me through finding myself again.

She is my childhood friend who has seen me through my darkest of times, literally helping me bathe and go to the bathroom while in a body cast.

She is my faithful friend as she let me go when I chose to go to college out of state.

She is my adventurous friend who moved to the big city with me after college.

She is my humble and forgiving friend as we survived a terrible falling out.

She is my family as we have survived tragedy together.

She is my fellow warrior in fighting for her family and understanding the difficulties of infertility.

We've survived distance of all kinds to only come back together because of our own individual struggles.

The unspoken shame. The impossible decisions. The heart stealing and soul crushing losses. The life long costs of IVF.

Only to strengthen this lifelong friendship.

And, then she asked me to be in the delivery room to coach her, along with her husband, as she delivered her first daughter. There were only tears of joy as I realized I would be there for that magical moment to see one of our chosen children take her first breath.

It has been an honor to walk beside her through this journey of life. I am immensely thankful for our bumpy path as it has prepared us for the brutal survival of our own battles with infertility. And it is truly with a full heart that I look forward to this next chapter of seeing her become a loving, and oh so grateful, mother.

I guess there really is only one thing to say to her.

Thank you… for being a true witness of me, for always seeing, knowing and loving me.

And, thank you for allowing me to be along for your ever upward.

Celebrating to Embrace Jealousy

The commercials start airing early to remind us all to get the perfect gift for some of the hardest working people on earth; mothers. I assume I don't have to go into exactly why Mother's Day tends to be difficult for us women who are childfree whether by choice, chance or circumstance.

As a woman who can't have children, seeing these commercials or hearing my loved one's Mother's Day plans is some of the, thankfully few and far between, times I feel my jealously come up. Admittedly, it is scary and difficult to even type that sentence.

Throughout my work of recovery I have come to understand jealously a little differently. It first started at the Emerging Women conference last October in Boulder when I saw an interview with Tami Simon and Alanis Morissette. Tami interviewed Alanis about the book she is writing and about her work with Relationships First. One of the points she spoke about was what she thinks the difference between jealousy and envy is. She said that jealousy is about connection; that when we are jealous of someone or something it is about self-improvement, we want it too. But when we are envious of something we not only want it for ourselves but we want to take it away from the other person, making it not about connection but disconnection. She used a really simple example of her hair. She said something to the effect that she knew many of us in the audience were jealous of how great her hair looked (it was the shiniest most beautiful head of hair I'd ever seen). She said that some of us were probably jealous of it (for sure!). She said we just wanted some of the hair gods to shine on us too. So her suggestion was to go out and buy the pomade she used to make it look that gorgeous. She then explained that if we were envious of her hair it would be more about chopping it off her head for ourselves so that not even she could have the luxury of her beautiful mane.

This definition makes sense to me. And, by this definition, I am jealous that the majority of women get to be mothers and I don't, but I am not envious. I am sure of this because it is one of the best parts of my life, and of my recovery, to see my loved ones be mothers.

And yet, I will admit feeling this jealousy doesn't necessarily feel good either. Through my recovery I have found that there are times I need to allow myself to feel sorry for myself and to feel that jealousy. To ask the impossible questions of why didn't I get to be a mom? Why does she? To feel that jealousy consume me, especially around the holidays or the first days of school or any other popular put your kids on your social media wall day. Don't get me wrong, I love seeing these pictures and posts and it isn't uncommon that I am showing your adorable children to my friends and family but I would be lying if I didn't admit that when I only have dog pictures to post, even though they are literally the cutest pups ever, my green eyed jealousy monster definitely rears it's ugly head.

But if I allow these thoughts and feelings to overtake my light my recovery suffers. For me the only way through this jealousy, to embrace and truly own it, has been through celebrating. I didn't know I was celebrating until a client of mine told me about one of her church small groups where they talked about celebrating as the cure to jealousy.

That's exactly what I do, I cure my jealousy through celebrating the very things I so badly want for myself in others. I surround myself with my chosen children because through this celebration my jealousy wanes. I ask to be as involved as much as possible in my friends' parenting and in their childrens' lives because through this celebration my jealousy loses some of its negative power.

This concept is not easy, but it is very simple.

And, for me, it works. Celebrating through my jealousy provides me with what life is all about, connection. Sitting in jealousy doesn't feel good and celebrating others' happy feels pretty amazing, simple but not an easy choice but a choice nonetheless. Besides, I know that my mom friends can sometimes have some jealousy of what my childfree life provides me.

If we aren't careful we can all get tripped up on wanting what we don't have and staying stuck in jealousy. And while, I will always suffer the lifelong losses and costs of infertility and my childfree life, I am also learning that I have some amazing things to be thankful for only because of this very bittersweet journey I have been on.

I don't want to be angry or envious, so I will allow myself to sit with jealousy but just for a bit. Then I will take that breath, find my gratitude and celebrate through to embrace it because only then do I honor my truth.

Scarred But Never Closed

Singing my heart out, holding back tears, as this seems to be what I do lately in church as I am wrestling so much with myself, with trusting and my faith journey, I had one of my first true writer moments. Smack in the middle of the song, I grabbed my bulletin and pen and wrote the title of this post and a line from the song down.

The song: Let Our Faith Be Not Alone by Robbie Seay.

The lyrics: "May our hearts be not of stone, give us souls that never close".

As a therapist I hear terrible things every day from my clients. And, it is not unusual for the thought to cross my mind that someone has every right to stay sick, to stay angry, to have hearts of stone and closed souls after what they have been through.

After infertility and the lifelong losses of three babies, I have also felt as if I have three very good enough reasons to allow my heart to become stone and my soul to close.

But I am learning, this is not meant to be the end of my story. Nor do I want it to be the end of my story; just as I help my clients every single day to make sure that their losses, traumas and tragedies are not their endings either. Because, I also get to hear amazing stories of hope and recovery every single day.

But this recovery requires the choice to choose hope *and* to do the work.

I will always have the soul scars of infertility and losing my babies. And if I am not careful these scars could very easily harden my heart and close my soul to the amazingness that is this life. As they are forever scars much like the four inch back surgery scar I have. Except, my soul scars are invisible to the outside world, and many times are completely misunderstood, invalidated, minimized and sometimes even ignored.

Either scar, back or soul, if ignored by me only worsens; the scar tissue building up, increasing the pain and decreasing my quality of life. For my back it is only through my physical therapy, exercise and self-care that this old injury and scar tissue can be as healed as possible. Nothing I do will ever make that scar go away but I sure as hell can make sure I do what is in my power to make it as better as possible. And, almost 20 years later, I wouldn't want that scar to go away anyways as it is a constant reminder of how much strength I truly hold.

As for my soul scars, I must do much of the same work. If I do not do the work of recovery from the trauma of infertility, the lifelong losses and costs of IVF and the ongoing work of accepting a childfree life, I will only allow the scar tissue to grow. And if I am not careful my heart and soul will scar over leaving room for only bitterness, anger and sadness.

Our trauma, tragedies and losses (infertility related or not) make us who we are. I have learned that I am a better *everything* because I wanted and loved those babies so much. I am also a better everything because I lost them. Sure, the losses left my heart and soul shattered at first, but now with daily work in recovery I have a scarred but healing heart and soul.

Scarred but better and complete, and most definitely open.

This openness is not possible without the daily practice of recovery, authentic living and courage. My choices in recovery, in daily practice, and my faith are what are required for me to not allow the scar tissue to close everything. And I did not survive infertility and lose my three dreams to only be left scarred, closed and hardened like stone.

I am still wholeheartedly figuring this whole thing out, awkwardly stumbling through this life in recovery. And, sometimes I am not a very pretty picture while doing it. What I think I am finally coming to terms with and learning is that I can trust that the end of my story isn't supposed to be a heart of stone or a scarred, closed soul. That I can trust my faith, doubts and all, because within this journey I will always have Him. And it is with His acceptance, love and help that I will continue to fight for, find and redefine my ever upward.

Change the Why

Why? The word that so many toddlers torture their parents with as their curiosity about the world overwhelms them so much that they must know why about everything.
Why? Why? But, why?

It is counseling 101, and in reality, one of the most helpful communication tools I teach to my clients. Take the why out of your conversations, especially the difficult ones.

Saying why can feel accusatory, and when we feel accused our defenses go up which means healthy communication typically becomes even more difficult and can even shut down.

Why did you do that?
Why do you feel that way?
Why do you think that?
Why can't you just be better?
Taking the why out of these questions feels a lot different.

What was that about?
How come you feel that way?
What is that thought process about for you?
What is holding you back from changing?

These small changes may seem trivial but just try saying those statements out loud to yourself and feel the difference. Now imagine how much your communication can be helped if you become more conscious of the why.

But, the why I really want for us all to change is your self-talk why. The why you beat yourself up with when you make a mistake.

I first learned of how hard I am on myself when I took a workshop with Kristen Neff, author of *Self-Compassion: The Proven Power of Being Kind to Yourself*, at Emerging Women last year. In the workshop, she talked us through her self-compassion break meditation and for the first time I had to see in my own handwriting how hard I am on myself when I make a simple mistake. That berating self-talk, calling ourselves names and really just not being nice to ourselves at all. This kind of self talk does not motivate us to change even though we've convinced ourselves that it has. We must realize what our inner critic is really trying to do, which is keep us safe or keep us from suffering or improve us but through the years it has developed a pretty mean way of doing so.

Neff's research shows that self-compassion is where confidence and change can really occur. Her self-compassion model includes self-kindness (talking to yourself like you talk to a loved one), common humanity (reminding ourselves that everyone struggles and everyone makes mistakes) and mindfulness (being present with all our emotions). Combine that with the shame resilience skills from the work of Brené Brown and your self-talk becomes a lot more pleasant and motivating.

A typical day for me will always include a trip, a spill or something breaking. It is just who I am, I am usually going too fast and as a firm believer in the one trip that often times means I am falling or breaking something. Yesterday for example, at coffee with a new friend as we are deep in great conversation I pick up my coffee cup to take a drink and it literally exploded; lid pops off, hot coffee all over my dress, the table and in my bowl of oatmeal (in my defense the barista had bent the cup before handing it to me but I was also moving too fast as usual).

Before learning the work of Kristen Neff and Brené Brown my inner dialogue would have been:

You're such an idiot. Oh my gosh, you are ridiculous. Why can't you be more careful? Just f*cking slow down! You're so stupid. How embarrassing!

After doing this work in my recovery:

Well, that had to be hysterical. That sucks, I'm covered in coffee. I need to stop, slow down and be more careful. Great girl, but not great choice.

I think we all struggle with this mean inner dialogue from time to time. I see it every day with my clients. What would it be like, how awesome would the world be, if we were all just a little nicer to ourselves? What if we took the why out of our self talk and replace it with how come or what? And finally, to do the work to remember we are worthy, lovable and great people who make mistakes but we don't have to be those mistakes.

The Complicated Gray

Several days after one of the most difficult days of the year for me, Mother's Day, I am reminded at how complicated this whole thing actually is...infertility, childfree living, loss, trauma, tragedy, faith...life.

I've written it many times before; life is hard and people are complicated. It never seems to be very black or white, which sometimes would be nice and so much simpler.

All of life is in the complicated gray; always between the simplicity of black or while. Nothing is ever all good or all bad.

It is all a beautiful complicated gray; especially when we give ourselves permission to feel it all, all at the same time.

This weekend I felt everything. Mother's Day was a good day but it was still super difficult and felt very sad, at least inside my own head and heart. All the talk of mothers and mothering at church wasn't easy to hear. Feeling torn and like a bad daughter and daughter in law because just acknowledging the day is difficult. However, I really needed to honor my own pain and myself. We also spent the afternoon swimming and playing with three of our favorite little boys which filled every cell of my body with pure joy, love and laughter. I was also so thankful for all the messages and cards I received and for the blogs I read about how wonderful and difficult Mother's Day can be for so many of us.

The complicated gray.

Our losses, traumas and tragedies are never uncomplicated; infertility, IVF and accepting a childfree life are definitely not an exception to this complication.

For me, especially as a therapist who has survived infertility and has fought to thrive thereafter, the complicated gray is always there.

The complicated gray I feel between the lifelong costs and losses of infertility and childfree living with the peace, freedom and happiness I have achieved through my recovery.

The complicated gray of making my almost enough moments my enough moments.

The complicated gray of honoring my losses but never allowing my heart and soul to scar over and close.

The complicated gray of the anger and bitterness at the unfairness with the trust and faith in the 'I'm okay and it's okay'.

The complicated gray of owning my shame and sadness while also educating and fighting for my story and the importance of my message and voice.

And for the many women out there struggling with any difficulty in the department of mothering and infertility, the complicated gray is never ending.

The complicated gray of living in shamed silence of infertility and desperately wanting and needing to be seen and heard.

The complicated gray of self-sabotaging ourselves because we feel so damaged and shamed in our infertility battles; betrayed by our bodies, by science and, sometimes even ourselves or our loved ones.

The complicated gray of every impossible decision that must be made in the journey of infertility whether emotional, financial, moral or ethical.

The complicated gray of every parenting decision.

The complicated gray of the cautious hopefulness and the reality of the statistical un-success of infertility treatments.

The complicated gray of our real stories not being seen, heard or understood by many.

I always work with my clients on finding the middle, seeing the gray and not thinking in such black or white terms. For the most part, our health and happiness lie in the middle; in this gray.

Through my infertility journey, my recovery and my ongoing acceptance of a childfree life I am learning that maybe we really must also truly embrace this complicated gray.

Because, I think, it is within this complicated gray we will find our permission for it all.

Permission for our stories.

Permission for our recoveries.

Permission for our light.

Permission for finding and defining our own happy ending.

Not Just Another Birth Story

Had our IVF worked with our surrogate Michelle, I would have gotten to be in the delivery room to see our babies be born. But that was never my path to experience. I sincerely thought the only births I would ever see would be the ones in that terrible 5th grade sex education class we all had to take and the sensationalized ones shown on television and in the movies.

So, when my oldest friend, my true witness of 30 years, asked me to be one of her delivery coaches when she delivered her first baby I cried with tears of honor and joy.

My friend who has seen me through my darkest of times and literally helped me through life in a body cast when we were much to young to handle such difficulties.

My friend who also knows the pain and losses of infertility.

My chosen family who I love so dearly.

Last week my friend gave birth to her daughter and I had the honor of helping her through her difficult delivery and being a witness as their family grew by one beautiful baby girl.

It is with much excitement and love that I (and her parents of course) welcome Abigail to the world! And with a full heart, I write her these words to hopefully last her a lifetime.

Dear Abigail,

Your mom and I have been through 30 years of friendship. We have been through things that really no two friends should ever have to see within a friendship. Your mom helped me through some of the hardest times of my life. I am sure we will one day share with you the stories of how she used to care for me as my nurse as I suffered through two back surgeries and lived in a body cast. She loves telling the stories of her helping me go to the bathroom, as I will admit they are pretty hysterical.

And on the day you blessed us all by coming into this world, I helped your mom through your very difficult and scary delivery. So, I now have my own stories to tell of things I simply can never unsee.

And yet, it was one of the most magical days of my life, as I know it was for your mom and dad.

Abbie, your mom and dad fought so hard to bring you here. Through three years they fought through frustrations, waiting games, anxieties, medical procedures, terrible side effects, misunderstanding from loved ones and the public and, especially, their fears; all to receive you.

Your mom and dad continued this amazing fight through their difficult pregnancy and on the day of your mom's labor and delivery, their fight only continued.

Scared of my own limitations, fears and queasiness I pushed through to allow my anxiousness to become excitement and I fought alongside your mom and dad. I fought for them and I fought for you.

I was so proud and honored to be there supporting, helping and distracting them throughout your mom's labor.

But mostly, I was so proud and honored to simply witness them in their fight. Your mom's diligence in containing her anxiety and fears for your safety. Your dad's advocacy for you and your mom's care and safety. And, especially their ownership in how you came to be whenever any doctor or nurse asked about you.

Simply, profoundly and wholeheartedly, I am just so proud of them.

We all worked together as a team to bring you into this world, your mom definitely doing the hardest work of all. And at 4:40 pm you finally graced your mom and dad with the joy they've been fighting and hoping for for three long years; your peaceful and perfect face, your dark hair and your healthy cry brought tears of joy to all of us.

Throughout your mom's labor, of almost two full days, your mom and dad lied to me about your name, even though I asked them a million times (as you will get to know I never give up easily). Finally, the morning after your birth, when your mom was feeling better, they gave me the best surprise of my life, your name. I was truly surprised and completely honored to learn your name is Abigail Justine.

It is with a heart full of love and honor that these are my promises to you, Abigail Justine, my namesake:

I promise to always do my very best to be that person your parents believed in and loved enough to name you after.

I promise to always be here for your mom and dad, for whatever they may need.

I promise to always be here for you, no matter what.

I promise to always be your soft landing spot but to also always guide and push you when needed.

I promise to love all of you, always accepting you and honoring you; with me you will always be seen, known and loved.

Because being there with your parents throughout their journey to conceive you and being able to be present for your entrance into this world is my ultimate enough moment.

Because you, Abigail Justine, are my ultimate ever upward.

With much love,
Your Aunt Justine

Seared Dates

I am a numbers person.

No, not the add, subtract, divide and multiply numbers kind of person (just ask my accountant husband).

The kind of numbers person who remembers dates, phone numbers and birthdays pretty well and for a very long time. I have clients' phone numbers committed to memory, for no reason, as I no longer work with them and my cell phone remembers them for me. I also usually, and very easily, remember birth dates of friends, family and all the chosen children in my life.

I also have many dates throughout the year that are forever seared into my very being.

I have always known the power of the dates that will haunt us forever as I often remind my clients of this. It is not uncommon that we begin to struggle some; anxiety is higher, depression is heavier or we just start to feel off and, when we stop to think of the date, or the time of year, and are reminded of that loss, trauma or tragedy that happened way back when.

I too have these kinds of dates seared into my heart and into my soul. My soul scars that never go away and in some ways haunt me all throughout the year.

August 25th, 1994 ~ My first back surgery.

June 19th, 1997 ~ My second back surgery.

December 28th, 2011 ~ The first phone call that stopped our lives, Michelle, our surrogate, was not pregnant.

April 16th, 2012 ~ The soul crushing and clarity providing phone call that our second, and last, embryo transfer did not take; Michelle was never going to be pregnant with our child.

June 26th, 2012 ~ The day we made another impossible decision to let go of our Maddie. The day of my true rock bottom.

August 31st, 2012 ~ What would have been the birth day of our two embryos transferred in the first round of IVF.

December 21st, 2012 ~ What would have been the birth day of our last embryo transferred in the second, and last, round of IVF.

June 17th, 2013 ~ The birth of Tipton, our chosen family's wonderful surprise, our bittersweet reminder that is outweighed by the love we have for another of our chosen children.

I wish I could have been better prepared by the infertility blogs, message boards and even doctors that these dates never leave us.

Especially, the birthdays of our never meant to be babies, at least never meant to be in our arms on this physical earth.

They are forever, for better or worse, seared in my head, on my heart and within my soul.

Today, I am able to say for the better.

And, through the work of my recovery I am beginning to have more of the magical, full of love, moments seared into every piece of me.

On June 22nd, 2014, I publicly declared the private decision I was finally able to make for myself on May 6th, 2014.

I was baptized.

Just a few days shy of my rock bottom when we lost Maddie 2 years ago, after surviving IVF and losing 3 babies, I walked into the waters of baptism that night a renewed, a redefined and a continually healing woman.

I walked into those waters with a scarred but never closed heart and soul and, with my three babies and all of heaven pausing to rejoice another sister in Christ.

On May 6th, my prayer that Jesus would show His love to me in a way I could finally understand, embrace and accept was answered. As I have written before, there is nothing like being a mental health therapist for over 16 years who cannot have babies to make one doubt God and struggle with faith. But, what I realized on May 6th, is that I can still doubt and question. I can even still hold feelings of anger and feel like my life hasn't been fair.

And, I can still believe.

Doubt, questions, anger and all.

Wonder.

I can believe in His love for me. I can trust His plan for me. I can live my life knowing the ending of my story will be

His way, whether or not I get to know it on this side of eternity. I can honor that He will take this life and let it shine.

My heart is full. My soul is continuing to heal. My ever upward wonder grows.

Seared dates, soul scars and all.

It is this wonder, my wonder, that makes it faith to begin with.

Our Infertility Rap Sheets

Ever Upward is growing. My world is expanding. My recovery is strengthening.

Which also means my shamed silence is triggered more often. Even though my shame resilience has grown as a result of my practicing recovery and the work I do with Brené Brown as a Certified Daring Way™ Facilitator.

As I meet more and more people in the infertility world, blogging or otherwise, I am finding myself comparing my story to theirs. I have always been uncomfortable with the TTC (trying to conceive) timelines. I am especially uncomfortable when our *About* pages and Twitter bio's are only our TTC timelines full of numbers and acronyms.

What I have come to realize is that my discomfort is simply a result of my shame being triggered.

The numbers we share to describe ourselves; how many miscarriages, cycles, IUIs, IVFs, BFNs, etc. seem endless. Hell, I had my numbers in my bio (two rounds of IVF and three never to be babies) when I first started writing. I thought I included these because they are part of my whole story. But what I think I am figuring out through working my recovery is that I have left them in for proof and as a way to cope with my shame.

Proof that I too have suffered and lost; my comparing my story to others', my way of shouting loud enough for all to hear, "I tried too."

My attempt at jumping up and down with my arms waving above my head while I shout, "I am here too!"

But, this really comes from my sense of not feeling enough, of trying to prove myself rather than owning myself. The scarcity culture, as Brené Brown describes in The Daring Way™ work. The never _____ enough. Never pretty enough. Never thin enough. Never rich enough. Never happy enough.

This scarcity culture has helped turn these numbers into one of my biggest shame triggers.

My fear that I will be judged that I didn't try enough. That I didn't lose enough.

Because I don't have a long rap sheet of years of trying to conceive or IUIs, IVFs and BFNs.

And, I have no doubt that I have been and will continue to be judged for not trying more, just as much as I am judged for not choosing adoption.

And so, at least from *Ever Upward*, the blog, I have removed my counts, my proof, because I am more than just my two rounds and three lost babies. I am actually even more because of my lifelong losses. These numbers could never come close to describing what I have been through or what is left as a result.

Because within this I truly own it, and myself.

Apart from surviving infertility and thriving thereafter, I also have the mental health therapist part of my head and heart at work with these TTC timelines and rap sheet descriptions. I cannot help but be scared and saddened by it. That as men and women suffering through infertility treatments we are identifying ourselves, sometimes completely, through how many treatments we have endured.

We are so much more than this.

We have to be so much more than this.

We have to be because that is the only way we will survive infertility and thrive thereafter, no matter what our ending looks like.

I am not sure what our motivations are for making our infertility rap sheets part of our bios or even our whole story. But for me, it was about comparison and scarcity. Comparison in making sure the world knew I tried too and therefore have suffered.

Scarcity in proving that it was enough.

Comparison and scarcity; two things I am practicing shame resilience and recovery from.

Because, I did try and I have suffered.

Enough.

Because, only I define my enough and my "did we do everything?"

For me, I need to be more.

I will talk about it, I will embrace it, I will practice and model recovery from it and I will own it. Because maybe within my ownership, one person will be brave enough to demand to be more than their infertility rap sheet.

Because we all are.

So much more.

And, we all deserve to be.

Defining Our Enoughs and Everythings

Amy Klein's post *You've Done Everything You Can* for the *New York Times* was the first spark I needed to write something about our enoughs.

Our enoughs and everythings.

When I wrote Our Infertility Rap Sheets, I was scared to death to put it out there and click publish. But, the feedback I received was the second spark I needed to write something about our enoughs and everythings. It was a message from a fellow warrior and blogger that ignited the third spark. Her bravery in reaching out was enough for me to pull this post from drafts, assign my own photo and share. As, she was in the midst of defining her own enough is enough and her everything.

As I have written, I've taken out my counts; how many rounds of IVF I tried because I have found I included them only out of my own shame. Out of this need to prove to the world, and maybe to myself on some days, that I too have suffered and lost.

Infertility or not, we all must define our own enoughs and everythings.

Have you done everything you can? Have you done everything you need to?

Have you done enough? Have you lost enough? Have you suffered enough?

Defining our enoughs and our everythings in order to let go, embrace and move forward.

I think we can apply these questions to many areas of our lives that we are struggling with.

Infertility. Recovery. Relationships. Dreams. This list goes on and on.

I think what we all must remember is that only we can define what is everything and when enough is enough. When we define these through others' expectations or society or because it is "what we are supposed to do" it only comes from this place of shame; a place of not honoring ourselves. Our enoughs and our everythings can, and need to, only be defined within ourselves.

If I don't hold on to this, I can very easily get wrapped up in the shamed silence that surrounds my infertility journey and my recovery. Because, technically, I suppose, we could have kept trying. Technically, science has provided many options for us to keep trying. Technically, there are also other options.

But to not listen to myself, my husband and our truth would have been the biggest disservice to me, our marriage and, in reality, to the world. For us to go above and beyond what we know is our enough and our everything would have destroyed us because it simply would not have been our truth.

We tried. We tried more than we had planned to. But, we tried again because our losses felt that crushing. We tried again because we knew that our everything wasn't met yet. Only we could make that decision. We need to explain it only to each other.

Only we define our enough and everything.

To let go of comparison, especially in our sufferings and recovery, is to find our truth.

Because we all suffer. We all lose. Hard is just hard.

And, we all must practice our recovery.

Trust in your truth. Trust in your everything. Trust in your enough.

Because, within that trust you will be found.

A Thistle of Dichotomy

It was a weekend of life's brilliant dichotomy for me; the complicated grey; the bad with the good, the dark with the light, the thorn with the beauty.

I'm not sure any woman enjoys their yearly exam at the OB/GYN but Friday was my day.

I spent an hour waiting in the waiting room with only parenting and pregnancy magazines to read with no cell service. And, a few uncomfortable pregnant women as my company (who I feel empathy for in their discomfort, jealousy toward their blessing in becoming a mother, all combined with a tiny piece of pissed offness and *are you serious God*??).

Once back in the exam room I can't help but laugh as I try to fit my ass in the paper drape left on the exam table for me (which I have never quite figured out how to use). And, despite being the healthiest I've ever been my curves still rip it almost completely in half.

Then the actual exam, no explanation needed, it is just the bad, the dark and the thorn.

Then the good, the light and the beauty as my doctor actually spends time with me. She truly believes in my story and is excited about the book and the blog, *Ever Upward*. I feel like an actual person with her and not just the woman who can't have kids.

The dichotomy continued with my kid filled weekend.

The bad, the dark, the thorn is having to be around a child that is very difficult for me. All wrapped up with the good, the light and the beauty in people who believe in my story, my progress and my message. All to come home to three of my chosen children spending the night with us for the first time for what is sure to be the first of many fun slumber parties; they are the good, the light, the beauty. Quickly followed last night by a pregnancy announcement that feels unfair; the bad, the dark, the thorn.

What I am figuring out is that this ever upward recovery I fight to live every day will always be filled with the dichotomy of life.

The good comes with the bad. The light comes through the dark. And many times, beauty comes with a thorn.

We don't get one without the other.

And thank God, because it provides us with immense perspective, gratitude and our truth.

There will be days where shaking off the bad, the dark, the thorn just really isn't that easy. I will admit I worked hard to shake it off all weekend. But, what I really needed was to allow myself to move through it all.

Because, sometimes, we just have to sit with it, move through it and allow it to pass. Trusting that if we do this work the good, the light, the beauty will quickly follow.

After all, this is exactly the truth and the light of ever upward.

Sometimes I need the reminder too, to which life and God will always provide, usually in the not so subtle smack upside the head for me.

The moments of the bad, the dark and the thorn make the moments of the good, the light and the beauty even more amazing.

And so, I will breathe it all in, embracing and trusting it because I know it is my authentic truth and because it is the only way through to my ever upward.

A Buried Treasure

The house had a seashell room.

The entire ceiling of a bedroom was decorated with a mosaic of seashells and mirrors.

Picture frames made of shells.

Lamps filled with more shells.

Glass tabletops filled with even more shells.

Then we found the moldy boxes full of seashells, at least four of them, buried in the basement.

They loved seashells.

As we cleaned out the house, we threw them all out, along with their years of painful hoarding and our years of three lost babies and a lifelong dream.

And yet, we see seashells every day.

And, I feel my lost babies every day.

The shells continue to come up in two different parts of the yard; emerging every time we plant or we get a heavy rain.

Like reminders of the past that will always be there right alongside the hope of what is to come.

And, my scarred heart and soul ache and yet, feel whole every second of every single day.

Both like a buried treasure, that isn't worth much and yet is a constant reminder of the past.

Just like every day moments or comments in my life that are constant reminders that I will never be a mother; will never quite fit in, will always be considered not whole, will always be judged and pitied.

Because, I am not a mother with living children.

And yet, I am more whole than I have ever been through my recovery from infertility.

Just like the every day reminders that I must practice my recovery: working on self-care every day, reaching out and asking for help, doing the things that help keep me healthy and practicing courage, compassion and connection. Because, I am recovering from infertility, scarcity, comparison, anxiety and depression.

And yet, I am whole in my practicing recovery from these, and from myself.

Our buried treasures of our past, of our losses, traumas and tragedies, will never stay buried forever. We will always have emerging seashells in our lives.

I guess this is where practice comes in. We must practice to use these reminders for us rather than against us. That they are not there to haunt us forever. But, rather to remind us of where we've been and how far we have come.

Within the buried treasure we can find our whole.

Within the buried treasure we can embrace it all.

Within the buried treasure we can be found.

Because, the buried treasure of losses, junk, gold, seashells and all, is our story.

Our story of the work of recovery.

Our story of the work and practice of our ever upward.

Loss is Loss

The loss of an eight cell embryo.

The loss of miscarriage at 6 weeks, 10 weeks, however many weeks.

The loss of stillbirth at any week.

The loss of a toddler.

The loss of any child.

Loss is loss.

I had the honor to process this lesson of life with a client on the same day that my fellow warrior at My Perfect Breakdown wrote a beautiful, kind of rebuttal, piece to my piece *Our Infertility Rap Sheets.*

And, again I am reminded that there simply are no mistakes made in this life or coincidences. And, that I have amazing people around me in this journey.

In her post *My Perfect Breakdown* discussed how her numbers are important to her because they are her children lost to miscarriage. In my piece, I wrote about taking my numbers out because, for me, they came from a place of shame, scarcity and comparison.

It is simply impossible for me to live a wholehearted life with courage, compassion and connection when I live from a place of shame, scarcity and comparison. I believe this to be true for all of us. And, I challenged those of us with the struggles of infertility to ask themselves where their count, their infertility rap sheet, was truly coming from.

What I did not write in *Our Infertility Rap Sheets* was the number I will never remove.

Three.

To the general population they may have just been three eight cell embryos.

To me they are my three babies.

My three babies who never had the chance to take a breath of this earth's fresh air.

My three babies who never grew.

My three babies I can parent only from this side of eternity.

My three soul scars.

My three.

Three will never be taken out of my story. It is within these three lost souls that I have been found and have found myself.

I see three everywhere I go. I feel my three every single day. I dream of my three and mourn the what ifs. I heal from losing my three always.

Being able to process this difficult lesson of life with my clients; women who have had miscarriages, women who have given up their child for adoption, clients who have lost their child beyond way too early to tragedy is something I feel honored with and thankful for.

Does is hurt less that I lost mine before they could grow?

Does it hurt less that she didn't suffer?

Does it hurt less that she was only in the first trimester?

Does it hurt less that I have lost three but she has lost five?

Does it hurt less that you at least got a couple of years with him?

Does it hurt less that she lived a longer life and mine never grew?

This comparison; this *my pain is worse than yours*, or even *my pain could still be worse*, is heartbreaking, soul crushing comparison.

And, it keeps us alone.

All alone with only our losses by our side.

If we can embrace that loss is loss; if I can sit across from my clients in the presence of their loss, with their loss, rather than comparing our losses then we are simply two mothers who have lost.

People who have lost.

And, that it is all just really fucking horrible.

But, we're in it together; at least, not sitting in it all alone with only shame, scarcity and comparison as our comrades.

Because hard is hard, hurt is hurt and loss is loss, and when we stop comparing we're in it together.

Isaiah

My friend and fellow warrior over at Rejoice,
Beloved reblogged one of my posts and in a comment she
wrote she led me to some clarity.
	She pointed me in the direction of Isaiah 54, and in
those words of scripture I found another piece of my soul.

ISAIAH 54
*Sing, childless woman, you who have never given birth.
Raise a joyful shout, you who have never gone through labor...
	Enlarge your house. You are going to need a bigger
place; don't underestimate the amount of room that you'll
need. So build, build, build.
	You will increase in every direction to fill the world...
	Don't be afraid, for there is no one to shame you.
Don't fear humiliation, for there is no one to disgrace you...*

	She wrote that my ever upward is my joyful shout to
the world. And, in reading her words I felt myself give myself
the permission I need to really fill the world with my singing.
	To build, to fill the world.
	To walk straight through my fears.
	This light inside of me to speak, to educate, to help and
to give myself and others permission.
	Permission to speak our truth.
	Permission to embrace our whole story.
	Permission to practice our recovery.
	Permission to own it all.
	Ever upward is my joyful shout.
	Ever upward is my mark on the world; my legacy, not
left in the legacy of my own children, and still my legacy.
	Ever upward is my continued seeking and fighting to
reveal our shame and rise above it.
	Ever upward is my connection to my story and to our
story.
	Because our stories, our shout or whisper to the world,
is the light and the love of ever upward.

When We Become a Mother

A deep knowing breath.
The warmth of a soul scar healing just a bit more.
A sense of truth, understanding and validation.
This is just a tiny sense of what I felt when I read these words from Lindsey Henke in her Still Standing post.

"But in my opinion a mother isn't born when a child is born. A mother and father are born when the dream of a child is conceived."

There are times when I allow my comparison, scarcity and shame to dim my light and I am fearful of sharing my story. This fear is born out of the messages my inner critic tell myself. The messages that have actually been said out loud to me. And, the messages that society drills into me.

There will always be some who will never ever consider me a mother. The ones who say I didn't try enough. The ones who judge my decision to not adopt. The ones who say I must not have wanted to be a mother badly enough. The ones who say I didn't lose because our three babies were only eight cell embryos.

I will never get full understanding from everyone, let alone validation. But, I will still speak my story. I will own all the parts of my story. And, I will continue to fight and break the shamed silence that surrounds infertility, miscarriage, infant loss and recovery.

But, I will not do so to convince my deniers.

I will do so because if I don't I simply am not living my truth.

If I don't I am not practicing my recovery, that I fought like hell to get to.

If I don't, I am not following my light.

I became a mother the minute I posted my ad on the surrogacy message board. I became even more of a mother when I met Michelle our surrogate for the first time. I became even more of a mother when our embryos were transferred into her loving and mothering uterus. I became even more of a mother the days we received the call that none of our babies were strong enough to even implant.

I am a mother with empty arms here on this earth. I am a mother who parents her children on this side of eternity. I am a mother to many people and things in my life.

Simply, I too, was born a mother the day I dreamed of becoming one.

I am a childfree not by choice mother who lives a child*full* life.

This is me.

This is my light.

We will dream and then sometimes we will lose.

We will suffer and then we can rise.

We will struggle and then we can thrive.

These are choices we must make each and every day. These are my choices to let go of what was never meant to be mine and to make sure it wasn't for nothing. Because I know I am a mother and more.

These are our choices to embrace our stories, to redefine and own it all.

This is life.

It is sad.

It is amazing.

It is ever upward.

A Letter to the Girl Trapped

August 25th, 1994 I had my first of two back surgeries, both of which left me in a body cast for 6 months following each surgery.

Twenty years later these are the words I need to say to that part of who I am still to this today.

The words to that scared 14 year old girl because in these words I choose to heal her.

Justine,

I know you are scared, but relieved that you finally have an answer to your pain. This is not the only time you will feel this gut wrenching and breath stealing bittersweet feeling. You will again feel this painful clarity on the day you receive the phone call that your last round of IVF did not work and you learn that your journey to have children is over.

But I can promise you, it is all worth it and you will be okay.

You have many years in front of you of struggle. A struggle mostly to find and believe in your light again. Because today, unfortunately, you will lose the biggest part of your spirit, only to fight for and find it again in twenty years, and only after devastating loss.

In twenty years time, you will find this light again when you have survived failed IVF, lost three babies and fought for your recovery back to yourself.

This event of your first back surgery, yes honey, I am sorry but you will have to survive another one of these, puts in motion everything that will make you an amazing being.

You will have incredible stories of inspiration and laughter to share with the world of your back surgeries. You will have incredible stories of struggle and hope to share with the world of your fight to become a mother. You will have incredible stories of loss and purpose to share with the world of your ever upward journey to find yourself and recovery.

You will come to understand, accept, embrace and own every part of yourself and your story. You will own your shame surrounding infertility by understanding how alone you are about to feel throughout these surgeries. You will have endless help throughout these surgeries; people who love you, even those who barely know you, will step forward to help in some way. Twenty years later you will have the language to understand that your light was lost even within this amazing help because it was given through sympathy and not empathy. Because, really how else does anyone feel but sorry for the 14 year old having to have back surgery, live in a body cast and miss half of her freshman year of high school? Let alone to then have to do it all over again in a few years.

Twenty years later you will have the clarity to no longer dim your light around your story of surviving IVF and accepting a childfree life because of pity. And, instead choose to shine the light to break the silence of struggle and hard.

Because sad is sad and hard is just hard.

Some things just really can't be fixed that easily; like a 14 and 17 year old in a body cast and a 34 year old woman who really wanted to be a mother but can't.

Find the joy and the love in the help from everyone around you throughout this time, even it if is only in sympathy, because it is still born out of the intention of great love.

Trust that you will thrive through this and that this isn't the end of your story; because, I promise, it is not even close.

And try, to hold onto that light just a little, knowing and believing that someday it will flicker again.

I promise this tiny belief and flicker is enough to get you through.

Because, your light will never be fully suffocated as you have an unending, ever growing and truly ever upward resilience.

In ever upward light and love,
Me

Choosing to Be Remade

I am not one to believe in the mindset of victim.

I do not believe we are victims unless we choose to be.

Labeling myself as a victim only leaves me powerless in changing my life.

Horrible things happen to all of us, hard is hard and struggle is struggle. If I sit in the victim place, at least for myself, I sit in the shit. Rather than being mindful of my suffering in order to move through it and then rise above it.

This has always been a common theme in my office, and probably always will be. I have said these sentences too many times to count, over and over:

You can choose to be your past.

You can choose to be your past mistakes.

You can choose to have all of your past hurts, losses, traumas and tragedies be your whole identity.

Or you can choose to learn from your past and move forward.

Or you can choose to embrace your mistakes and try again.

Or you can choose to make your past hurts, losses, traumas and tragedies just a piece of your story and not your whole identity.

You choose.

So it isn't surprising that when I heard the song *You Are More* on Joy FM by Tenth Avenue North I was immediately sending it to some of my clients. The chorus goes,

You are more than the choices that you've made,

You are more than the sum of your past mistakes,

You are more than the problems you create,

You've been remade.

I realize when the artists are singing, *you've been remade*, they are referring to Jesus dying for our sins and with this grace we are remade. But as a mental health therapist, even one with my own strong, and yet questioning and always wrestling faith, I must meet my clients where they are, faith or not.

Even with my faith, and the amazing grace of Jesus, I think, I also must still *choose.*

We must choose to be more.

We must choose to be more, faith or not.

And if Jesus isn't your thing, well, then you still have a choice to make. You can choose to be more than the choices that you've made. You can choose to be more than the sum of your past mistakes. You can choose to be more than the problems you create.

You can choose to be remade. You can choose to not be a victim to your life circumstances, your past hurts or mistakes. You can choose the power to change your life.

Choosing to be remade is my work in ever upward. When I choose to be remade because of and within the grace and love of Jesus, but also because I choose every single day, I choose me. I choose to be more than the woman who cannot have kids. I choose to be more than the woman who survived infertility and lost three babies. I choose to be more than depression and anxiety.

Because we are so much more than those past choices, past hurts and past mistakes. They are just pieces to that brilliant life puzzle, they are pieces of our story. We must do the work to embrace them all.

Because only then will we own all the parts of our story.

And, only then do we choose to be remade.

An Imposter

They turned up the lights after one song.

We usually sing four amazing rock band like songs which is one of the many reasons I love our church.

Then I remembered seeing the reserved seats walking in, "Reserved for families of children dedication".

Shit. Oh, shit.

Today is the children's dedication at church.

Okay, I can do this. I can hold it together.

I can celebrate through my jealousy and focus on the love of these families. I can focus on how adorable these kids are and how much their families love them.

I can do this. I can do this.

Nope.

Pastor Greg asked all the supporting family to come and join the families getting dedicated up front and we bowed our heads in prayer.

I have no idea what was said, at this point I was trying to focus on keeping my breathing steady in an attempt to not break down in heaving sobs.

Amen.

Lights dim, the singing surges back up and I sit my ass down to sob.

It's been a while since it has hit me like that; like a two ton boulder sitting on my chest, like the rug of life being pulled out from under me, like a swift and stinging smack across the face.

And like everything else in my life, especially my life as a recovering therapist, it is nothing short of extremely complicated.

Ever Upward was launching in just a couple of days. A book that at first included *to Own a Childfree Life* in the subtitle before I changed it to *to Define Your Own Happy Ending.* A book where I write about my struggle through infertility to accept a childfree life and thrive thereafter.

And yet, there I sat sobbing in the dark after the children's dedication at church that morning.

Do I still have a ton of work to do?

Should I be able to handle this better by now?

Should I not be even more saddened as I hear my parents sniffling beside me knowing that I will never be able to give them grandchildren from Chad and I? Or are they sniffling just because they can see how much I am hurting?

Should I not be angry that families like us are not mentioned at all? And, that we aren't even the tiniest glimmers in anyone's heads or hearts?

And yet, can I still be so thankful that many won't even have to think about living life without children or won't ever have to pursue infertility treatments or lose babies?

Should I not be even a tiny bit cynical that infertility has changed how I see the world forever? As I looked at that line of families and asked myself in my head which ones suffered losses before, which ones had to use fertility assistance, which ones are still hurting just like me.

Am I a fraud?

Or am I just human.

An always grieving, yet healing, mother with a scarred heart.

A mother with empty arms on this side of eternity.

Can I be sure of my messages and advocacy in *Ever Upward*, can I own my acceptance of a childfree life, and still be healing and hurting all at once?

The release of my book doesn't mean I have this all figured out, I have never once claimed that. But what I am coming to understand is that it does come with this fear that people will think I am okay, that I am healed, that it doesn't hurt anymore.

Overcoming the Lifelong Losses of Infertility is the first part of *Ever Upward*'s subtitle and those words were chosen for very specific reasons.

This will always be hard. This will never go away. It lasts a lifetime.

There will always be those days that it hits me out of nowhere, like today. There will also always be those days that I know will be hard, like the due dates, every single year. There will always be times of the year that it feels impossible to be a part of social media. There will always be the reminders that I don't quite fit in.

The struggles and the losses of family planning are never forgotten and I think, maybe never even healed.

But, I must choose to be forever healing.

I also must trust that this isn't for nothing. That I have not suffered these losses for naught.

It is through this work I can make sure that I am healing, that I am recovering, that I am scarred but never closed.

Ever upward isn't always easy but it will always be worth it. And this means giving myself permission to sometimes feel the world in my losses but to feel it in my enough.

And, so I choose; I choose to embrace that I will be a forever healing and grieving mother.

The Most Ironic Story

It was a full circle weekend for me when I returned to the Emerging Women conference, this year in New York City.

Last year I attended EW as a woman shrouded in self-doubt and cloaked in the darkness of shame.

A woman who had lost. A woman who had fought for recovery. A woman on the edge of figuring out what to do with that tiny spark inside that she knew meant something.

I left EW last year with the spark I needed to finish writing *Ever Upward* the book, start my blog and continue to walk into and fight for my continuing recovery.

This year I walked into EW as a woman more motivated than ever (sometimes to the detriment of my recovery), shining bright with the spark of recovery, ownership and true ever upward light.

I mustered up the most bravery I have ever practiced and handed, maybe even forced fed, my book to the women I admire and who have inspired my work. I practiced valuing my work both through confidently selling it and through allowing everyone to see how much it means to me and how much I believe it can help.

I left the conference with a plan, with motivation and with more connections than I ever dreamed. And yet, I left the conference knowing that I will always be this very messy work in progress, practicing recovery daily and working to own all the parts of my story.

And, as usual life made sure to remind me of the irony of moving ever upward; this dichotomy of life.

Chad joined me in the city for a few days following the conference as we had never been to New York City. Late Monday night we decided to attend the Today Show on the Plaza. Which meant the alarm went off at 5 am to get in line.

What did we have to lose? We could, in the least, get the beautiful cover of *Ever Upward* on national television. And maybe, just maybe, Matt or Natalie would notice it and take a few copies (especially to give to Bobbie Thomas).

We go there early enough for the perfect spot, right on camera when the hosts come out to shoot.

Where's the irony?

To our left is an adorable couple from Florida with a sign, a bright pink and blue sign... *We're on our babymoon!!!*

My heart skips a beat, I hold my breath and feel the thorn of shame.

To our right is a group of ladies celebrating their 70th birthdays. One notices my book cover and asks about it. I give her my sales pitch about what *Ever Upward* is, to which she replies that all three of her daughters went through IVF and one of them is actually adopting at the end of the month. She says how impossible it all is (even the adoption part) and how sorry she is.

Okay, this is my little miracle. I was totally meant to give this woman a book, she gets it.

And, then she blurts it out, "Well, why don't you guys just adopt?"

Shame doesn't overtake me completely this time and I take the chance to educate her on fertility compassion and also remind her of how difficult she just said it is. She mumbles something and proceeds to literally turn her back to me for the next hour. I hear her whisper to her friend parts of our story, including the words, "Well they should just adopt if they really want kids that badly."

I literally feel the shame oozing from her into me.

My heart skips a beat, I hold my breath and feel what now feels like the sword of shame.

Here to promote my book and I am between the couple who is on their babymoon and the grandmother who gets it but is still judging me harshly.

Before the shame can completely crumple me to the ground, the hosts all come out to say hi, Matt, Natalie, and Al. I'll admit I am a little starstruck as I have been watching Today since I was a kid. They are all very kind and genuine as they shake your hand and say hello.

Then you see all their eyes notice the beautiful monarch butterfly on my book cover; all three hesitate to take in the beauty. Then the magic happens, Natalie asks about it and even takes a few copies and promises she will make sure Bobbie gets one.

I can't believe it. We are so excited, so too are the couple and the grandmother for us. You see, even though my dementor of shame tried to make me think these were the hardest three people for me to stand next to, they were actually my miracles for the day. As I gave them books the couple admits that they started trying because so many of their friends have struggled with getting pregnant and their doctor recommended starting immediately due to age. I looked at them with just the tiniest bit of jealousy but mostly I just felt love and excitement for them. The grandmother said she was excited to read the book and share with her daughters. I replied that I hope they enjoy it while in my head saying to myself that I hope she really enjoys and learns from Chapter 3-Owning Adoption.

Life is ironic. And it is never a mistake.

Sometimes it knocks me on my ass at first but I will always choose to move ever upward and see the love, the connection and the miracle that is meant to be.

As incredible as my trip to NYC was through the learning and self-growth, the friendships, the vacation and the acts of courage I never thought I was capable of it could have never prepared me for the most ironic part of this ever upward journey.

Thursday I was visited by what I choose to believe is one of my never to be babies, perhaps it was just a butterfly regardless she came to deliver the magic.

She came to remind me of myself.

She came to love me, as she stuck around for several minutes and let me get super close to her.

She came as a sign of ever upward.

Because just over an hour after her visit, one week after I left for EW and my NYC vacation, I had my first piece picked up and published by HuffPost. I have worked, tried and submitted for almost a year to be picked up by HuffPost. It took these failures, these lessons, along with the spark of magic, connections and courageous motivation from NYC for it to actually happen.

My post was run by HuffPost Parents.

This childfree, yet child*full*, mother is officially a HuffPost blogger.

A HuffPost Parents blogger with two pieces published in two days.

Full circle moment?
Nope, she told me it is just the beginning.

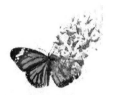

Part II

Year 2

The Warm Embrace

I am practicing my patience, some days with gritted teeth and total white knuckles, but I am actively practicing it trying to relax in the hammock (I explain below I promise). The patience I need as *Ever Upward* gets into the hands of those who need it, is seen by the eyes that need to read it and is felt by the hearts that need the connection of it. This sometimes painstaking patience is lit up by the messages and reviews *Ever Upward* is slowly receiving.

Ever Upward is a book of my story. My story through the losses of infertility. My story into the acceptance and ownership of a childfree life. These words had to be on the cover because I trust the infertility community to help me get the full story out to the rest of the world. But they were also words we thought about leaving off the cover because Ever Upward is so much more than an infertility story that ends in owning a childfree life.

It is a book about life. A crazy epic story about overcoming the hard stuff and finding and fighting our way to being okay; to being better than okay, even when life didn't turn out how you hoped, dreamed, planned or paid for.

I want this book to be the permission we need to talk about our stories, the permission to embrace them, the permission to fight for our recovery and our version of the happy ending, and most definitely, the permission to own it all.

I hope people fighting their way through the darkness of infertility treatments find comfort in my words.

I hope people trying to figure out what happens next when it didn't turn out how they hoped find their way in my words.

And, I hope anyone struggling with the darkness of life finds the light they need in my words.

What I was not prepared for was the messages and reviews from mothers, mothers of all kinds; mothers to living children, mothers to angel children, mothers to living and angel children.

Me, the woman who cannot be a mother, the woman who wrote a book with the term childfree in the subtitle, is being lovingly embraced by the very club she will never be a member of.

And, yet it feels like home.

A home we all belong to.

Because, somewhere along the journey of surviving and thriving this life and especially in the making of our family, we have all lost and suffered somehow, somewhere.

Because it is not a club of just mothers. It is a club of anyone who has struggled, lost and survived.

So, a club we are all members of.

Because, when does life ever really turn out how we had planned or hoped?

And, yet we can do this work.

We can choose to be okay.

We can choose to be better than okay.

We can find our ever upward.

This surprising acceptance, this warm motherly embrace, has left me finding even more ever upward in this journey. This wholehearted embrace by the very group of women that I may forever long to fit into has allowed me to let this all be just a little bit more this week.

Or as my therapist helped me with my metaphor in letting this be…I think I am actually sitting in the hammock.

Let me explain.

The endless work of the last year or so are the fishing poles I have cast out into the crystal clear turquoise water. I must stick those poles into the warm white sand of the beach and walk away. They are cast to the big fish that could easily change my life and show the world *Ever Upward* with one tiny chance they give me. They are cast to every single person who needs to give themselves permission to find their own ever upward. They are cast out to you. And, I must stop putting my toes and hands in that beautiful water and allow it to become that crystal clear calm glass so you can be drawn to the amazing light that is this work. So, I am actively working on walking away, grabbing my sangria (served in a carved out pineapple of course) and sitting in that comfy hammock to soak up the embracing magic of the sun and of my own light.

This is how the perfectly imperfect person I am is going to muster up the strength to let this be, trust the work I have done, trust the universe and get the hell out of the way.

Sitting in the hammock, soaking up the sun, breathing in the salty air, sipping my sangria and truly allowing myself to really receive that warm embrace from the club I'll never belong to.

Making It Well

One of those Sundays in church that you weren't sure what you needed, if anything, but you get it anyways.

We all struggle. We all lose. We all will hurt.

And yet, so many of us are struggling to not only do the work to survive this life but to embrace that these struggles, losses and hurts can, will and must become well with our soul.

But, we cannot do this alone. I'd even argue to say that we cannot do this with only our faith either.

We need support. We need help. We need each other.

As Pastor Greg spoke about our struggles he discussed that God will often send Jesus in skin; the person we need to help us through the dark struggle. Pastor Greg went into a whole story about being with his family in an overwhelming and scary situation and how their guide was wearing a red shirt. God protected them and sent in a red shirt.

In other words, we need both spirit and actual being to help us through.

They closed the service with a version of the old hymn It Is Well with My Soul, and with the words let go my soul and trust in Him…it is well with my soul. I allowed myself to continue the work I have done in embracing the hard stuff. Everything I have survived, all the losses, is well with my soul. My story, my ever upward, both in my struggle and recovery and in my work of the book, blog and my private practice, allows me to help. Practicing the work of recovery means allowing it all to be well with my soul.

Not necessarily fair but well, okay, at peace.

That Sunday Chad and I just happened to sit behind one of my young clients and her family. After the song ended her mom turned around to me with tears running down her face and said, "You're our red shirt, thank you."

And, in that moment I felt even more clarity I didn't even know I needed.

That clarity where you feel with every sense of your being that you are experiencing a piece of your puzzle being put perfectly into its place in the beautiful picture of your life. The right time, the right place, the right people all put exactly where they are supposed to be for this unexpected, brilliant moment of clarity.

Sometimes these moments are shoved in our faces and hearts, sometimes we must be open enough to receive them, sometimes it is a little bit of both.

In her six words I felt God, I felt love, I felt the universe, I felt the light and my light.

I felt the forever scarred soul of who I am heal just a bit more.

I carried that into my sessions that week.

It is an honor and privilege to do the work I do. I love what I do. I love walking alongside people as they choose to change their lives. Sometimes, I have to push from behind and sometimes I pull from ahead but mostly I simply walk alongside.

It was with this clarity that I was able to be with a client as she told me she was pregnant after years of trying, as she struggled to say the words, struggling out of disbelief, fear, guilt and out of protection for my losses.

And, yet I was able to be her red shirt. Because I know she is only in my office because she had lost herself in her battle to make her family. Because I know I was only able to help her because I am the therapist I am today after my own losses. Because I know she will be okay no matter what because of the work she has done with me. Because she has given me the honor and the privilege to be her red shirt.

All of it, two back surgeries, failed IVF, lost babies, anxiety and depression is only well with my soul if I choose to do the work to make it so.

My choice lies in what I do with where I have come from.

My choice lies in the power of moving ever upward.

Out of the Ashes

One week shy of 9 months after my dad's life changing fall off a ladder, my family has faced another life threatening and forever life changing tragedy. I have spent the last week alongside Chad's family in Denver on another of the scariest roller coasters of my life.

There is no doubt that my dad's accident prepared me for this journey. I knew what kind of support my family would need because it was the support that I lacked myself during dad's accident. So I bossed; making people sleep, eat and take breaks. I counseled; providing the space to vent, talk and cry. I helped; starting the Caring Bridge site and simply just being me. And, I walked through it with my continually growing faith; allowing my in laws to give themselves permission to beg and question God for their daughter's life while also trusting Him and their faith. As my friend Kelly told me, I think I may have a calling as a chaplain in my future.

I may never get to know why this year has been both the best and hardest year of Chad and I's lives; a job promotion for Chad and launching *Ever Upward* for me, and yet we have also experienced these two family medical emergencies, that were literally life or death.

What I do know is that I felt different through this emergency, I felt my faith more than I ever have. I also witnessed too many miracles to ignore the fact that He does have a plan for us. And, even if in this moment I am not sure I like, or even want to accept, His plan, I still know that it is and will be okay.

I trust this more than I ever have in my life. I trust this because of my journey out of my ashes; two back surgeries and a year in a body cast, the lifelong losses of infertility, three lost babies and the rock bottom of my life. I believe, especially with having faith in something, that we can fight for and find our beauty out of the ashes.

There are many things I do not know. I do not know when my sister in law will get a new heart. I do not know how difficult this road will be for all of us. I do not know if Ever Upward will ever get the big break I so hope it does. And, I do not know when the next trauma, loss or tragedy will strike me or my family.

However, there are many things I do know. I know that we will be okay no matter what. I know that one day I will get the understanding of the why I so desire, even if it is just on the other side of eternity. I know that if we continue to give ourselves permission to talk about it, embrace it, practice recovery from it and own it all, we can all find the beauty we all so deserve no matter what we face.

This is the work of faith.

This is the work of life.

This is the work of finding and moving ever upward.

Forever Changed, Never Fixed

Surviving loss, trauma and tragedy means we are forever changed. Thriving thereafter means we figure out how to be okay. Finding and moving ever upward means we figure out how to be better than okay.

Things can and will get better but I am not sure we are ever fixed.

Just because the subtitle of Ever Upward included at first the words to own a childfree life and just because I often write the words acceptance of a childfree life does not mean that I am fixed.

Just because a woman gets pregnant after struggling to do so, whether or not through successful treatments or unexpectedly, does not mean she's fixed or all better.

Just because the adoption has gone through doesn't mean that the family is fixed.

Just because we have survived...

Just because we are putting one foot in front of the other...

Just because we seem or are better...

Just because we got the goal...

Just because we are done...

Does not mean that it is like it never happened or that we are all better.

We are doing the work.

We are forever healing.

We are forever changed.

But, never fixed.

When we have suffered through the difficulties of family planning, infertility or not, it comes with figuring out how to be okay with the lifelong losses; the scars. Even, when we determine what our happy ending is, it doesn't undo the painful journey we've traveled before.

Working with women through the infertility process has meant that I help them give themselves permission to feel the complicated grey of it all. Because, after suffering through any level of infertility a woman just doesn't get to be excited about finally being pregnant. Infertility steals this excitement and joy from us. And, what makes it even worse is when the people around us feel like we should just be okay or better or, worse yet, fixed.

Survivors of infertility know the millions of things that could go wrong, because they have gone wrong already.

Survivors of infertility know how quickly your joyful high can be crushed by the breath stealing loss of heartbreak.

Survivors of infertility no longer have the luxury of living in the black and white like a lot of us think, and even sometimes demand, that the world exists.

We've lived through it, felt it all and literally embodied the complicated grey that life really is. Nothing is all good or all bad. As a therapist I work a lot with clients on challenging the unhealthy thinking pattern of black and white thinking.

Life just isn't that simple.

Infertility or not, whatever we have had to survive in this life, and we will all have something, it is never I think, all good or all bad. And, I just don't think we have a choice but to be forever changed by it all somehow. This is the work we must do. The work to be okay; to be better than okay. Because, that is where our choice lies, to choose how to be okay after we've survived it.

To choose how we are forever changed.

Accepting and owning a childfree, yet child*full* life, does not mean that I am fixed. Losing my three babies forever changed me but it is within my power to choose how they changed me. For today, it is in finding my purpose to use the gifts He has given me. It is in giving myself and others the permissions we need to truly embrace all of ourselves. The permissions to make choices not through desperation or fear but through wholeheartedness and love. The permissions to determine when our enough and everything is.

To stop proving it. To truly own it. To break the silence. To embrace it all. Living wholeheartedly brave.

This is my story.

This is our story.

This is Ever Upward.

Living in the Tension

I cannot tell you how many times I have said this phrase in my office lately.

Another way to describe my concept of the complicated grey.

Because nothing in this life is all good or all bad, despite our brain literally being wired to over-categorize and to think in the black or white or in the all or nothing.

Life is simply just too complicated.

I believe our happiness lies in living in this tension between the two worlds; living in this complicated grey.

It is the best way to describe how my life and my recovery have been after surviving infertility and defining my own happy ending. I must practice this work of living in the tension because this recovery is complicated. It includes lifelong losses of the infertility journey. It includes managing, and therefore being a thriver, of anxiety and depression. And, it includes practicing the daily work to be better than okay.

As a mental health therapist I have heard the phrase it is what it is in many contexts.

Half of me believes this statement can be about acceptance. The acceptance of things that cannot be changed. The acceptance of our circumstances. The acceptance of what is not in our control. Many of us could be happier and healthier people with this work in active acceptance.

But the other half of me knows that this statement can also be used in an apathetic way. The way to declare powerlessness. The way to assume being the victim. The way to choose to stay stuck, stand in our own way and not change our lives.

Recovery for all of us must lie in the tension between active acceptance and this passiveness. In other words, perhaps we must work to find our place between the two; *to embrace that feeling lost between the two just may be where we find our magic; where we actually find ourselves.*

At least that is where I have found mine, as it has only been in embracing this tension that ever upward was born within me and is my love to share with the world.

The work of living in the tension between overcoming the lifelong losses of infertility and defining my own happy ending.

The tension between the sadness of not being able to be a mother and the freedom and joy of being a child*full* mother.

The tension between the days that the sadness, anger and unfair bitterness strikes and the days I know I am okay, actually better than okay because of this journey.

The tension between soul crushing sadness and emptiness and the deep knowing breath of my version of mothering.

The tension between the hard anxiety and depression days and the choosing to practice recovery from both.

The tension between feeling alone in the pushing and delivery of *Ever Upward* and trusting that God has it all in His hands and perfect time.

The tension between never fixed and forever changed.

The tension between knowing what I know and trusting what I can't.

The tension between soul scars and always healing.

The tension between accepting what is and hoping for what could be.

The tension between the struggle and the choice to practice recovery.

The tension between doing and letting it be.

The tension between fighting until our enough and everything and never giving up on ourselves.

Simply, and yet utterly complicated, it is the tension of our brutal and beautiful lives.

Because, it is within this tension, and the complicated grey, that the brilliant colors of ourselves, and of life, emerge; embracing that within this tension our ever upward will be born.

Through the Darkness We Can Awaken

Every day I help people through the toughest times of their lives. Every day I model the work I teach. Every day I challenge and comfort. Every day I teach and sometimes even beg.

Everywhere I go I am asked advice. Everywhere I go people often feel comfortable enough to tell me their deepest darkest struggles. Everywhere I go I see people searching, seeking and fighting to find more happiness in their lives and trying to figure out how to be more whole.

We will all have to eventually do the work to be happier and healthier versions of ourselves. We will all have to embrace our lives, get out of our own damn way and own all the parts of it. We will all have to love ourselves enough to choose to change.

And, without a doubt, especially lately, I am learning this work must include taking care of ourselves. It must include the self-care part of our recovery, the self-care part of our lives.

No matter what your darkness may be; there is never dark without the light. At times in our lives our darkness may be our current circumstances, in which case we do the work to remind ourselves that this too shall pass. At times in our lives our darkness may be our haunting past, in which case we do the work to heal, let go and choose how we are forever changed by it. All the time our darkness can easily drown us and forever change us for the worse if we allow it.

What I promise is that the dark only gets darker and lasts longer unless we choose to do the work. What I promise is that there will be days that being awake can feel beyond vulnerable and downright brutal. But, what I can also promise is that they will be the best days of your life.

Lately, the difference between the times when I am in the dark and doing well and the difference between my clients that are greatly struggling in their own darkness and the ones who are saying to me, *"I am finally awake"*, is a lot of self-care and a lot of choosing to do this work.

This brutal, hard, frustrating but amazing work of recovery. Especially, the self-care part of this recovery. My clients who are looking at me with engaged eyes and love for themselves are the ones who have trusted me enough to try to choose to love themselves just a bit more by practicing self-care.

The self-care of making time for ourselves. Practicing daily routine. Eating, sleeping and moving better. Looking inward through prayer and meditation and presence. Truly practicing self-compassion. Bravely creating. Using our words effectively. And, beginning again when we mess it up a bit.

This is not easy work, but it is very simple.

I simply choose my self-care every single day.

I simply choose to move through the dark in order to shine.

And, I will challenge, comfort, model, beg, teach, love and help until you simply choose it too.

Moving Through Not Fitting In

Many of my closest friends have not had to think about their fertility much. They began trying, they conceived, had relatively easy pregnancies and deliveries and, best of all, have allowed me to be a part of their growing families.

Then there are my friends who have struggled in making their families. They know the two week waits, the lifelong losses and heartaches and the financial and emotional consequences that seem to last a lifetime. But even still, they were able to have the children; the traditional happy ending.

Then there is me.

Sometimes that sense of being different than every other woman in the room can feel like it is literally taking my breath away. The sense of not fitting in can feel especially difficult when it catches me off guard and is during a time that I am so grateful for.

Chad and I spent the weekend out in Vegas for our goddaughter, McKinley's 2nd birthday. We love spending this time with my friend Casey and her family, as we are so thankful to be a part of McKinley's life. She quite literally is the brightest ray of sunshine and fills my heart and soul up so much, I am so blessed that she is one of our chosen children.

And yet there I was at her 2nd birthday party where every other woman there had at least one child or one on the way, feeling like I was the last kid called to join the team. Watching Mac play with all her friends was so much fun but not knowing many of the other guests very well left me observing from the sidelines; which as a therapist, I'll admit, is honestly one of my favorite things to do.

But then it settled in, that nagging you are very noticeably different than all these women. You do not have anything to contribute to these conversations.

And I struggled.

Fuck.

It bothered me.

It bothered me way more than I wanted it to or expected it to.

I soon realized, I also did not have my usual back up. When I am around mothers who know me well I do tend to be pulled into the motherly conversations most simply because of what I do for a living. I realized this weekend that the fact that I am a therapist, and that it is so much of who I am and not just what I do, has been a saving grace in this lifelong recovery from infertility and living a child*full* life. It is a saving grace because my professional opinion is often asked and the parenting I do with my clients is often recognized. That and I have really amazing friends who respect my opinion and love me well.

What I think I am learning now is that I need to believe in this part of my parenthood as much as my closest friends do. I need to believe in it enough to show myself and others that I too fit in, even at the 2 year old birthday party with all the other mothers.

Because I have a lot to contribute.

Because I do belong.

Because I am a parent.

So much of this lifelong recovery of thriving after infertility is our own work. I cannot say how long that twinge of feeling like I don't fit in will last, maybe forever. But, I do need to acknowledge that it is up to me to trust that I always belong and to believe in my own worthiness as a parent in this world.

My Christian Complexity

I am a Christian. I curse…a lot. I have tattoos. I believe in the power of love and connection. I believe in the Universe. I am afraid and brave all of the time. I doubt and question a lot. And, I believe.

The equinox is here on March 20th 2015 and a powerful portal is opening up with a total solar eclipse and New Moon in Pisces on the same day!

What does this means exactly. As I have read and been told by some of my much better educated in this realm friends, it means rebirth and starting anew, a reset and the power to get it all done!

Sounds like my kind of magic and exactly what I (and we all) need.

But I had to ask my friend Kaeleigh, "But what does that mean for me?"

To which she reminded me that I am pretty aligned with these things and making the world a better place. But, I had to push her.

"But what can I do?"

I mean, I'd like to capitalize on this too! *Ever Upward* could really use this power right about now!

And her response seriously made me laugh out loud.

"For you oh, Christian magoo, I suggest meditating and maybe a vision board."

I love it. She's right, how does one combine this kind of thought with their Christian faith?

My self-care includes practices such as yoga, meditation, tapping and believing in the power of the Universe. This may make some Christians cringe. But, when I refer to the Universe I believe the Universe was created by God. And yes, Jesus is my Savior.

Can I hold onto these truths? I think so. I mean life is hard and people are complicated. And, thus you have the complexity of me. As I think we all are. Just as I told one of my clients today as we were discussing God, life and recovery; do what you feel drawn to, what works for you and give yourself permission that it doesn't necessarily have to fit in one box.

Be fully you, in all her complex glory.

I responded to Kaeleigh that this Christian needs some fucking star power, pixie dust, unicorn glitter and magic too. And, so I meditated (as I do every day). And I prayed. And prayed. And prayed some more. And read some scripture. And, I made that vision board, filling it with hopes, dreams and realities. And, I've decided to share it with the world because then it is like planting it in the fertile ground to grow strong roots toward the ever shining sun.

The Completeness of Just the Beginning

On Friday I was surprised by an email from the Barnes & Noble in Saint Louis where I will be doing my first book signing with an incredible picture of my book on the shelves!

There she is, my baby, on the shelves of an actual bookstore.

I literally gasped with tears of joy.

As I have come to expect of life, my life especially, there will always be joy right along the struggle.

That night Chad and I attended our first class of a marriage seminar our church offered. I had requested to not be seated with couples who had young children for obvious reasons. We sat down and directly across from me was a woman who was about 6 months pregnant.

I looked at Chad and whispered, "You've got to be fucking kidding me."

Yep, I totally said that in church.

Then we learned the couple next to us was also expecting, 11 weeks along.

I took a breath, held back the tears, looked up, said a quiet prayer and said out loud, "Challenge accepted."

It was a great first class, I learned so much about what a healthy, biblical marriage looks like. I also gained a better understanding of Ephesians 5 which left me with an understanding where I do not gag on the word submit.

Class ended and I knew I had to face the pregnant women again tomorrow and I would choose to be okay. When I turned my phone back on I was notified that my Thunderclap campaign went through (thank you God) which means that over 91,000 people will be notified of the *Ever Upward* launch on April 7th. When I turned my phone back on, I was also able to read one of the most amazing reviews someone had posted on Amazon!

The dark with the light, the joy with the struggle; this is what you get when you choose to live an engaged, wholehearted courageous life embracing the complicated grey.

And it is worth every single second.

Saturday night Chad, my parents and my friend Lindsay ventured to the bookstore to see *Ever Upward* in person. We wandered together at first trying to find that beautiful orange breakaway monarch on the cover to no avail so we eventually we split up.

"I found it!"

I had shouted way too loud for a bookstore.

I stood there by myself for just a few seconds in this moment of awe; overwhelmed by a completeness and yet, the sense that this is really just being the beginning.

I felt proud. I felt accomplished. I felt happy. I felt deserving. I felt excited.

In that moment I allowed myself to feel all the goodness.

But, along with all that goodness also comes the reminder of the journey I had to survive to get here, the losses that have forever scarred my heart and the part of me that will always be different.

I am learning this journey never ends. I will never be complete or at the end of it; or at least in how I expected. It will only be through my own work and recovery, through my connections and relationships and through my faith that I am okay.

Just as I sang in church today, "I stand in Him complete." And so, even though I may never feel the completeness of finality, I know I can find it in Him. I know He has this; just as He has Maddie and my three never to be babies.

I know in Him I rise ever upward and therefore this is just the beginning.

Shifting the Definition of Success

She is out there; for all the world to love and judge.
She has been born; for all the world to embrace or reject.
She is shining bright; whether or not she sells or bombs.
At this point the making of *Ever Upward* has been years, and as of last week she has now been born into this big, scary and incredible world.
And, it feels awesome.
Saturday was my first book signing in a real book store. I went in with absolutely no expectations, or at least I tried as the very normal human being that I am.
I mean, no expectations = no disappointment.
Right?
And, just like everything else in this incredible journey, He had a lesson for me.
I had 20 people RSVP for the Facebook invite. The store manager at Barnes & Noble said that if I sold 10 books it would be considered a very successful signing.
Part of me me thought for sure this was doable. And of course, that perfectionist part of me desperately wanted those 10 sales, better yet 11!
But then there was reality. It was a super nice day in St. Louis on Saturday, which is sometimes hard to find in early Spring. I am a first time author. And, my book is about one of the most shamed and misunderstood topics in our society.
Shit, I'd be lucky if I sold a couple books. And 45 minutes into the signing, I had settled for selling just 1.
Panic did try to settle in off and on, especially those first 45 minutes.
But, I fought her off by choosing my perspective. I practiced gratitude.
I am an author. I am an author signing her first book in a real bookstore.
God, I am so grateful.
Of course, He quickly started showing exactly why I was there that day for my first book signing.
And, it was not to sell books.

For the record, I only sold 3 or 4 that day and only a few of those 20 RSVPs showed up.

I was there to connect and educate.

First, was the older woman who stopped by and told me about her grown children who went through infertility. As we chatted, she was adamant that they got kids though so they are completely fine and would not need my book. You can bet I took that moment. I pointed out that part of the title is Lifelong because the infertility journey changes us forever, even if you do get the happy, healthy kids out of it.

No sale but she promised to tell her kids about the book.

Next there was the woman who looked at me with the fellow warrior compassion and said, "I had to go through infertility too and it didn't work for me either." She then told me about her two amazing daughters she adopted from China. We talked about the child*full* life and the scars that the infertility journey leaves us with.

No sale but we connected as mothers, her as a mother to her adopted girls and me as a child*full* mother.

That perfectionistic panic and doubt tried really hard to take over here. If I couldn't get these two women to buy my book, then I did not stand a chance of making one sale today.

And then *He* gifted me the moment the entire day was for.

A mother and her three kids were lingering by the table, I smiled and said, "Hi!"

The mother then pushed the younger daughter forward and said, "She would really just like to meet a real life author."

My heart soared and I smiled hugely, "I guess that is me, I am a real life author now."

The girl, maybe 10 or 11 years old came right up.

"How do you exactly write a book?" she asked excitedly.

As I am telling her my book writing process her mom picks up *Ever Upward* to read the cover and the back cover, she lights up, "They're IVF babies!" as she places her hands on the tops of the girl's and her twin brother's heads.

She goes on to explain that they both know how hard mom and dad had to fight to get them and how they are products of infertility treatments. And then her eyes fill with tears as she realizes that infertility treatments did not work for me. I tell her that *Ever Upward* is about my journey, defining my own happy ending and how I live a child*full* life.

And, that I am okay.

The conversation continued with much excitement. I gave the little girl an *Ever Upward* journal, "For free!?!", she exclaimed. And she asked me to sign it.

I made her promise that she would write in it every day for at least 30 minutes because this helps our creative writing muscle grow. Her mom then explained that she would be homeschooling next year and she looked at her daughter and said, "Maybe she will be your English pen pal? Why don't you ask her?"

I of course said yes. As they walked away, I took that all familiar deep knowing breath and felt my soul settle, tears came to my eyes and I got it.

No sale but an amazing moment of childfull living.

I was in the bathroom when they were checking out with their other purchases, the little girl was upset when I wasn't at the table anymore. When she realized I hadn't left she ran up and gave me a huge, and quite possibly, the best hug ever. I reminded her to keep writing and to definitely email me.

I pray I hear from her and I pray her mom knows how much that moment meant to me. And best of all, I am so thankful that some of my closest friends and my family were there to share this with me.

I have always known *Ever Upward* was not about the royalty pay outs or the fame. But, society (and my own perfectionism) can really challenge this truth at times. I am thankful that through practicing my daily work in recovery, I was open enough to accept the gift of what my book signing was really meant to be for and mean; connection and education.

Doing this work allows me to be open to what He has in store for me, the true gifts. It is only through this lifelong work that I allow it to be good.

Better than good; ever upward.

She Rears Her Brave Heart

We are halfway through National Infertility Awareness Week (NIAW).

And honestly, it is kicking my butt.

Kicking my butt both as a survivor, and especially thriver, of the infertility journey but also as an advocate. This is living in the tension and the complicated gray of life, I teach this every day to my clients and life reminds me of it myself often.

As an advocate, I always shine the light on infertility and educate whoever will listen. I shout at the top of my lungs when it comes to spreading the healthier messages of infertility like: we must be more than this heartbreaking journey, the detriments of the 'never give up' message and that there are many versions of the happy ending.

This advocacy requires incessant sharing on as many platforms as possible this week. Because just maybe my story will reach the person who needs it most in that moment and they will know they are not alone. Because maybe my story will reach the person who needs to tell someone their story and ask for help. And because maybe my story will reach the person who needs to give themselves permission to embrace the complicated gray; to feel lost and confused while at the same time trusting that they do actually know what is best for them on this journey.

But, as the survivor and thriver of infertility, I am also a child*full* mother who infertility treatments did not work for. I am the child*full* mother who will be forever changed and have to work on always healing the scarred losses of her three never to be babies.

And, this survivor is honestly struggling, and ironically struggling with the theme of this year's NIAW: You are not alone.

Hope is a huge theme in the infertility world. But, as a mental health therapist and a survivor of infertility, I also know hope needs to be balanced with the work of active acceptance. Many of the stories being shared this week are stories of hope and therefore success. They are posts with the long laundry list of infertility treatments and ultimately with the socially accepted, most desired and traditional happy ending of a baby. All accompanied by the adorable and complete family picture.

My *story* feels nothing like these success stories; my family picture does not include babies, infertility treatments did not work for me, I am not adopting and am finding other ways to parent.

If I am not careful those differences can make me feel like I do not belong and feeling like I am alone. But I know and choose to believe that is nowhere near the truth. I know this isn't true because all of these success stories have also been difficult for some of my clients. Especially the ones who are embarking on what will be their last treatment and they are left feeling alone too.

And, this is where the advocate rears her brave heart.

This is why our messages in the infertility community must change and be healthier. We must stop comparing our numbers. We must speak that there are many versions of the happy ending. We must practice active acceptance. We must be more than the infertility journey and the quest to become parents.

And we must fight this together; not abandoning those still in the trenches, not casting out the ones who treatments work for or who choose adoption and not forgetting the childless.

We are in this together. And we are in it together forever, because these scars last a lifetime.

I am not alone and neither are you.

Let us thrive and rise ever upward together.

Shining My Faith Through Doubt and Wonder

My dad asked to borrow my bible, (The Voice version) to see if he likes it. I, of course, said yes when he noticed I had a bunch of papers stuck in it. I mindlessly took them from him and placed them on my meditation/prayer altar and did not think of them again until this morning during my prayer and meditation time.

One was a letter I wrote to God at the end of our church's Explorations class. Honestly, the class that changed it all for me. This is what I wrote one year ago to God and probably to myself all at the same time,

> *This has been some of the most challenging years of my life, which I feel like is saying a lot considering what I've already been through. And yet, I finally feel, not only more me, but I am finally feeling at peace with me, with You, with it all. I think I need permission to doubt and question, and then I really needed to admit that I was, and maybe still am, so angry at You for what I've deemed as unfair. And yet, I also know at the same time that I don't get that power of what is fair or unfair in this life, in Your kingdom or what You have planned for me. And more than ever before, with this knowledge, with this peace, with Your grace, I am finally trusting You. I feel this sense, Your spirit, inside of me; almost always. I'm still definitely learning and questioning and figuring out how to do this all, but it is with this sense of faith that I'm both proud and a little scared. But I also am going to give myself permission for that fear because I don't ever want to lose my wonder about this all or about You.*

A year has passed since I wrote these words and my sense of trust in them has only grown. This sense that I can stop treading water so hard all the time and know that His hands are underneath me to help me float. This sense that everything will be okay, even if I am not loving it all right now.

A year ago this week was when I walked into the waters of baptism and every day since has been full of growth and wonder. This coming weekend I will take part in my church's baptism services. I will walk on stage and share my faith testimony with our congregation of thousands. And, in front of those thousands of people my "cardboard testimony" will have the word infertility on it.

What I hope is that I give someone else permission to seek themselves through this journey of infertility.

> *To know that everything will eventually be okay as we define our own happy ending.*

> *To know that this journey has nothing to do with punishment or what is fair or unfair.*

To know that through embracing the complicated gray, they will actually find their truth.

My prayer is that in that dreaded, and yet now completing word to me, infertility, the hope of being okay can shine. And, most of all, that we all can trust that we can rewrite parts of our story, trusting in how He has it all in His hands, and that the end of our story is nothing short of a grace filled miracle.

Are They Thinking It Too?

A mini post about something that, of course, caught me off guard and has been bugging me a bit.

Do the mothers think of us non-mothers in a group conversation?

A few weeks ago I attended the biggest convention of my life; 7000 people big. Which means I met a lot of incredible people and I had to give my elevator speech of who I am many times over.

There is always that part…the part where you share about your family and my response is one not many people identify with, "No, we don't have kids, we tried but can't have them."

Sometimes the conversation ends there, sometimes they try to fix my pain and offer the usual quick fix of adoption and other times they lovingly want to know more.

But then as the weekend goes on and as I get to know these incredible women and am having so much fun the conversation inevitably turns to their kids and being mothers.

And I am left without the experience to contribute and completely in my head.

Sometimes I wonder, do they ever stop and think of us?

Do they ever have that moment of, *Poor Justine, we're just talking about our kids and she's over there and she can't have them.*

Or do they never have that thought and I am just personalizing all of it way too much?

But, I know I am not the only one out there who has felt this way. So my question, for our recovery, is what do we do with this?

I think our job is to make sure to stay engaged. If we disengage from the conversation completely we lose connection. And, we already feel lonely enough as women without children in our society. So we must engage and look for that moment to contribute to the conversation or maybe even change the subject.

Or maybe one day, we can brave enough to just call it out and just state the awkwardness that we are feeling, and maybe they are too.

What I know for sure is that I will continue this work in rising ever upward to always be engaged in my life, even when I am feeling that sense of not fitting in. Especially because, most likely, it is in my head and only my perception that is causing that feeling.

And that, is completely changeable and in my control.

Or Just Stand

I have been blogging for a year and half now. A lot of learning, growth, healing and connection has happened in that year and a half.

190 posts of learning, growing and healing to be exact. As I am continuing to work on growing the platform of *Ever Upward*, I am growing my YouTube channel. You can find Self-Care Tip Tuesdays, funny videos of the dogs, tapping scripts, my appearances on *Great Day St. Louis* and videos of me speaking to old blog posts, so please subscribe!

I originally wrote *Tread or Float* in February of 2014. This is a slightly reworked and updated version of it.

~~~

For the last 15 years I have had the honor of witnessing people journey through some of the most difficult times of their lives to emerge as happier, healthier and whole people. As a mental health therapist I fulfill multiple roles on a daily basis; teacher, healer, helper, educator, coach, big sister, mother, friend, confidante, trainer and, in all honesty, sometimes I'm the provider of a swift kick in the ass. Unbeknownst to them, my clients also, at times, fulfill these same roles for me as they are my reminders, and examples, of fighting the good fight to being better than okay.

Throughout the years of working with clients I have found there will be times where I must push, and I mean push really hard. Making sure they know they have the strength to change their lives; and that they are ready. There are other times where I will simply hold their hand, walking alongside them through their journey of self discovery, self doubt and finding peace. Then there are times, where I will take their hand and pull them forward, at times, begging them to trust me and try things a different way; to put one foot in front of the other and follow me.

No matter the concern someone is coming into therapy and coaching for, they are facing the hardest work of their lives. They are facing times of progress and times of feeling so stuck they can't stand it. They will doubt their abilities, and maybe even mine to help them. They will get worse before they get better. They will at times hate me for the things I ask them to do. They will walk away and come back. They will push me away because it hurts that badly to trust someone or to have someone believe in them so much when no one else ever has.

They will question.

They will resist.

They will work.

They will change.

Simply, we will all face struggle.

Where we lose ourselves, I think, is when we make these struggles *all* of who we are. We turn them into our whole story. They become our entire identity, even when they start working against us rather than for us. We hold on so tightly to these struggles and what we think works to manage them that we lose the great parts, the whole parts, of who we are.

When our struggles are our whole story, we struggle to own those stories, and therefore struggle to find our ever upward. We must find the way to make these struggles simply parts of who we are, parts of our story.

But we hold onto the trouble, the trauma, the loss, the struggle because it is all we have ever known. We hold on because the unknown is scarier. We hold on because we have no idea what else to do. We hold on because, at least we're surviving. We hold on because the old ways of coping have worked, we think they are our water wings, our life preservers.

But eventually, we hold on so tightly and so long, the very things that have saved us, that have helped us to survive, become our own cement blocks.

Our own cement blocks drowning us in ourselves.

What I ask my clients to work through and change every day is no less than an act of faith and trust. I am asking them to let go of their way. The way that has actually worked for years, at least worked in numbing or self-medicating themselves. The way that has helped them to survive but is now drowning them. I ask them to let go because if they don't they won't have any free hands to grasp onto the tools and the hope I am offering them.

They must let go in order to begin again.

But the most excruciating part of this battle, is that they must have faith that they will either float or tread water while they learn, grow and change.

Because they will. They will tread or float, and I will be right there with them; coaching, believing, pushing and loving.

And eventually, they will be able to grasp onto those tools.

But most importantly they will find their freedom to finally believe in the hope I hold for them.

And they will save their own lives.

They will find their own ever upward.

For me, I have also come to trust that not only can I trust and have faith in myself that I can tread or float but also there is a firm foundation just underneath me that I can trust. Reading one of my Sarah Young devotionals one night, helped me feel it completely. Just underneath me in the ocean of life, in the water that I may feel like it drowning me, are His hands.

I just have to stand.

At Peace Is Not Yet My Story

Surviving through infertility changes us forever.

Choosing to thrive thereafter simply means we figure out how to live the rest of our lives with our forever scarred soul, and yet do the work of healing every day.

A couple of weeks ago I participated in a faith testimony at my church. It was one of the most amazing experiences of my life. We each walked out on stage, in front of thousands, holding a piece of cardboard; one side stating our struggle and then flipping to the other side of how our faith has changed us.

My faith has been a significant part of my healing from infertility. Three years ago, I would have literally told you to fuck off had you told me that. There is not much like being a mental health therapist, who hears terrible things in my office every day, who struggled with infertility without the desired outcome, to make one really angry with God.

But here I am, attending services every single weekend, serving regularly and looking to start a faith-based infertility support group.

Here I am choosing to heal and making my faith a part of that.

As an advocate for infertility, I also knew I had to take part in the faith testimony. That is until, they wanted me to walk out on stage with the words "at peace" on my piece of cardboard.

Not a chance.

At peace, will never describe my lifelong recovery from infertility. And, I felt like I would abandon every single person in that congregation who was struggling or had struggled with the infertility journey.

Sure I have moments of peace. But part of my forever healing is living in the constant tension of accepting what is, practicing that active acceptance, balanced with the forever longing that I want to be a mother.

You can argue that we chose to stop treatments, that we are choosing to not adopt and that this means my longing has melted away with this acceptance. But our choice to not give up on ourselves, to know when enough was enough and to let go of a dream that was not meant to be ours was a choice between two not so great choices.

I am not sure any survivor of the battle with infertility would ever use the words "at peace" to describe their journey, their healing or their recovery.

I have two people in my life, who through a lot of work chose to also not give up on themselves. They decided to stop treatments and figure out what life could be for them living a childfree not by choice life.

And then they got pregnant. They will forever live in the tension of getting the happy ending balanced with the sense that they had finally let go of that dream balanced with the sense of whether or not to try for more.

This is the *complicated gray* of the joy of motherhood after being forever changed by the infertility journey.

I have people in my life who are struggling with secondary infertility. Who never had to think of ovulation kits or treatments for their first but now have had to go to all lengths to add to their family.

They feel so grateful for their child or children, but have always dreamed of having more. They will forever live in the tension of being grateful for what they have balanced with the guilt of wanting more balanced with the anger that it is just not fair.

This is the complicated gray of the joy of being a mother after being forever changed that they may be a mother to only one and not many.

I have many in my life who infertility treatments worked for. They got the 'successful', paid for and happy ending.

And yet, even they will have to figure out life with these lifelong scars that their family was not built in the easiest or normal way. They will feel grateful balanced with anger that it took what it did to get their family balanced with the fears and worries that infertility settles into your soul and mind forever.

This is the complicated gray of becoming a mother through the soul crushing war of infertility.

And then there is me. I've defined my happy ending, I live as a child*full* parent.

And, I am happy, honestly happier than I have ever been.

But, I am not sure I will ever be able to use the words "at peace" when it comes to my life without children. Infertility simply steals this from us. It changes everything, forever. The only way to have those moments of peace, the moments of clarity and truth that we are okay is through shifting our perspective and doing the work. The work of breaking the silence, sharing our story and finding the new version of who we are and who we want to be with these forever scars.

Simply, the work of choosing to rise ever upward.

The Accidental Farmer

To clarify, I am the accidental farmer.

To clarify more, I am the accidental farmer of monarch butterflies.

If you have read the book, if you have read anything of this blog or if you know me in person you know how much butterflies mean to me. A breakaway monarch graces the cover of my first book, I have butterflies tattooed on my body and Chad and I have worked very hard to plant 2 (for now) huge butterfly gardens on our Mason House property. The gardens of course include milkweed in our attempt to help save the monarchs.

The life cycle journey of the monarch in particular is miraculous and the perfect metaphor for rising ever upward.

On July 4th we had the honor of witnessing a monarch lay her eggs in our butterfly garden. It was one of those moments of awe and clarity. In my usual childlike wonder I kept tabs on the eggs and researched galore on what to expect. Well, I now currently have over 45 monarch caterpillars in an aquarium on my kitchen counter. In the last week we have witnessed them grow exponentially in size. Next week we will watch them climb to the top to form their chrysalis and then about 10 days later they will emerge beautiful monarchs.

Thus far we are in awe and complete amazement at these creatures. How beautiful they are, how fast they grow, what they have to go through to molt and grow bigger and how much they eat, which also means how much they poop!

To watch a caterpillar literally walk out of its old skin to grow bigger takes the butterfly metaphor even further than what is typically understood. The monarchs have been rising ever upward since the beginning of time.

Giving Ourselves Permission to Feel It All

Many of us are taught there are 6 basic emotions; happy, sad, anger, disgust, surprise and fear.

Part of my job as a therapist is to teach my clients that we were taught too simply, as there are many kinds of each of these six emotions. For example: there are many kinds of anger. Are you frustrated, enraged, pissed off, irritated, etc.? When we are able to accurately identify the emotion we are more equipped to cope with it.

What I have learned throughout my own recovery after infertility and now working as an advocate and helping many clients through and after the journey of infertility is that there is something even more powerful than knowing all the different kinds of emotions, how to identify them and therefore cope with them.

There is room for them all; room to feel them all.

Even all at the same time.

This is where the movie *Inside Out* nailed it brilliantly. Sadness and Joy can be felt all in the same moment, and for many of those moments it makes it even more amazing of a life moment for us. As I watched the film I prayed that every parent would see it and learn the message that we must feel the dark with the light, that there truly is room for it all.

Just be happy is not the answer to our problems.

But I also desperately need every adult, especially those going through struggle, to hear this message too.

We must give ourselves permission to feel it all; all at the exact same time.

Freedom with sadness.

Anger with joy.

Acceptance with longing.

Fear with bravery.

Contentment with sorrow.

Trusting with feeling forgotten.

Happy with jealousy.

Bitter with love.

For me, this is what I call the complicated gray of life. I think we must give ourselves permission to feel it all, to feel what we have been previously taught are opposite emotions at the same time. I think we must give ourselves this permission, because when we make room for it all we can find our clarity.

We can find our freedom.

I believe when we walk into this feeling of lostness, into the complicated gray, we make room for the light.

In this permission our magic can be born.

And, we can heal a little bit more.

Instead of our struggles leaving us empty bitter shells of who we once were, our permission to feel it all and to embrace the complicated grey helps us heal and leads us to the truth of who we are and who we want to be.

Feeling our emotions, all of them, especially all at once is messy, scary and uncomfortable. But, giving ourselves this permission is what will allow us to take the deep knowing breath and have the courage to take that one tiny step forward.

That one tiny step forward to who we want to be and who we are supposed to be.

The Post-It Miracle

My first book signing was back in April when *Ever Upward* launched. My first book signing was nothing about selling books, as I wrote I had to choose to shift my definition of success.

My second book signing was this past weekend, and as He would have it, was also nothing about selling books.

I had a short talk prepared, to which there was no one to give it to which only solidified my lack of expectations for this book signing. But, Chad and I made a day of it, we had already had a great lunch at a local place and enjoyed connecting with people we would have never connected with throughout the day.

For the record, I sold two books.

One less than my first book signing.

You see I don't have the big publisher behind me. I was just now able to invest in the literary publicist. And, my marketing plan for this first book has remained writing for free for other publications and working my job that pays the bills, seeing clients.

Publishing a book is not for the faint of heart. Publishing a book about a topic that no one wants to talk about, can at times, feel like career self-destruction. Let alone publishing a book about this said topic when your story makes the world very uncomfortable because you are not one of the success stories.

And yet, there is always something churning...

We may not have full understanding in the moment, but have faith there is always something amazing in the works for you.

So I did not deliver my talk and I sold minimal books, but it was the ending to the afternoon, just as with the first signing, that ended in a goosebumps kind of way.

In lulls of the two hour book signing I was reading Pam Grout's E-Cubed on my phone. I had just read my manifesting assignment for this experiment: Be a love bomber (leave post it's of love in random places around the world).

As we were getting ready to pack up and I was signing the remaining books we had not sold, Chad said, "That's weird, look there's a post it in your book." Then a Barnes and Noble employee said, "Oh, I found one earlier too!"

Two post-its with messages from only God knows who.

One read, "Stars can't shine without darkness."

The other, "Don't worry, everything is going to work out!"

In completely different handwriting.

It's a post-it miracle!!

Goosebumps, tears and gratitude along with the deep knowing breath in allowing myself to feel it all; fear of failure, stress that this will never get noticed, trust in knowing it will, belief in myself that it already is, and most of all, knowing trust in that it is all exactly as it is supposed to be.

Needless to say we went out to a nice (early bird) dinner to celebrate and toast our post-it miracle.

Honoring Them

Yesterday was one of our seared dates.

I was a successful normal person yesterday instead of an evolved therapist. I busied my way through the day keeping my mind off the date that will never leave me. Sure, I got a lot done and the things I got done bring nothing but honor to our never to be babies but I also know I must allow the sadness, grief and forever longing to be.

Because only through the darkness do we make room for the light.

And so, with my scarred but never closed soul I wonder who they would have been, I grieve the lifelong losses with both sadness and anger at how unfair it sometimes feels and I trust I am making them proud by how I parent them from afar and always choose to rise ever upward.

Hope

Hope can be a tricky concept for many us, especially those of us who have gone through any kind of major struggle, trauma, loss or tragedy in our lives.

I am a survivor of infertility and loss.

Through our infertility journey hope at times was our best friend and at other times was our worst enemy.

You see my faith did not grow strong until after our infertility journey ended. And you may be surprised, as our journey ended without the desired result of babies. I usually tell people there is nothing like being a mental health therapist who struggled with infertility to make you be pretty mad at God.

And yet, here I am, my faith the strongest it has ever been.

This strength was not found in hope, but rather in allowing myself to doubt and question. And yes, to even be angry with God.

It was within my doubt, questioning and anger, and allowing myself to fully embrace it all, that His clarity washed over me.

And hope shined again; a healthier hope that is.

Not the hope that if we kept trying, kept praying, kept doing what society told us to do that God would do our will because we had hope.

I had to learn to let go of this hope because if I am truthful it was only the hope for things to turn out the way I wanted; how I thought things needed to be.

It was the clarity of a healthier hope that came with learning to practice active acceptance of what we cannot change balanced with the trust that He holds the end of our story.

Within my working faith, within the doubt and the questioning, I allowed enough room for hope to be a true anchor.

We have this hope as an anchor for the soul, firm and secure. (Hebrews 6:19 NIV)

This work has allowed hope to be an anchor for my soul, not a hope for my plan, but the clarity and trust in His.

And, so I will continue to hold His hope for my life, even if it has not necessarily turned out how I planned.

Because, I know he has the end of my story, and I trust it is amazing.

Birthing a Rare Kind of Parenthood

It is not uncommon that an interview with Kim Cattrall be shared on multiple media outlets. However, it is uncommon when you consider one of the topics she discussed: how she parents even though she does not have her own children.

Across social media her quotes ignited comments of both major support and criticism. As an advocate for breaking the silence of infertility, pregnancy loss and recovery I was excited and as a writer, I have my own words.

~~~

I always knew my journey to parenthood would not be traditional, and yet I never could have imagined the unexpected extraordinary life that has been born of my journey.

I met Michelle on a surrogacy website. My husband and I were beginning the journey to make our family through gestational surrogacy. Michelle was a mother of two children and a first time surrogate. We did In vitro fertilization (IVF), putting both of our bodies through synthetic hormonal hell, transferred a total of three embryos, lost our three babies and our dreams to make our family ended.

Who are we if we are not parents? What is our legacy if no one carries on our family name, our gorgeous red hair, vivacious laugh and vibrant, passionate personalities?

Do I matter if I cannot be a mother? Do I dare speak out even though I am not one of the success stories? Do I dare ask you to listen? Do I dare stand here and parent?

In our world's most accepted definition of a parent, I will never meet the criteria. I will never birth a child and I am not adopting one. So you will call me childless. And, I will then emphatically and stubbornly correct you and let you know that I am a child*full* parent, birthing a rare kind of parenthood.

I will never get to parent the newborn narrowly missing the blowout diaper or experiencing the night of bonding while breastfeeding and rocking her to sleep. I will parent by holding whatever baby is available and helping whichever parent needs a break. I will never get to parent the first steps. I will parent the steps in helping someone change their lives for the better after trauma, loss and tragedy. I will never get to parent the first days of school. I will parent the teenager struggling with

debilitating anxiety. I will never get to parent and see what of me and which of my husband is in my child. I will parent to teach empathy and understanding of how hard it is to make a family. I will never get to parent the holidays; wrapping gifts, picking costumes or dressing them in matching outfits.
I will parent my growing faith; allowing doubt and questioning to only strengthen it. I will never get to parent through the graduations or the weddings. I will parent through modeling and teaching every single day, helping people to give themselves permission to be okay no matter how their lives have turned out.

Parenting is not about biology or even the status of having children, as there are many of these parents who parent less than I do on a daily basis. Parenting is about pushing from behind, walking alongside or pulling forward. It is about championing and advocating. It is about being able to see one's true light even when they are unable to see it themselves. It is about showing the way to walk into it all in order to embrace it and find truth and clarity.

Parenting is showing up bravely and loving with your whole heart. And, you're right I do not get to do that in your tradition definition of a parent but your perspective of my story does not change my truth. The truth that within my three never to be babies, I have fought for and found my ever upward in unexpected parenting roles; birthing a rare kind of parenthood, but a parenthood no less.

My Shifting Shadow

My trip to Montana for the Haven Writing
Retreat with New York Times bestselling author Laura
Munson was the best money I have ever spent, the best
moment I have ever listened to that voice telling me I have got
to do something and some of the best days of my life.
Montana is my happy place. Laura is my friend, coach
and a gift to the world and my life; I learned so much from her.
In addition, there simply are not enough words for the women I
met at Haven. They are my new found tribe that I so
desperately needed after the last year of lonely platform
building and trying to get *Ever Upward* noticed and selling.
They are my soft landing spot full of inspiration and love.
I found my voice there in the quiet of beautiful
Montana. And most of all, Laura and my new friends helped
me to discover that my passion, although one of my very
best qualities, was allowing the mission to get in the way.
And so, I am anew; practicing my art of writing
differently, and daily, and working on the sequel to *Ever
Upward* in a completely different way.
Because through only my truth and only my voice will
the mission actually shine bright.

~~~

And so, I thought I would occasionally share some of
my writing prompts that I work on daily here at *Ever Upward*,
especially while I work more on the second book for now. I
hope you enjoy, I hope they inspire you, I hope they make you
laugh, and most of all, I hope you can trust me in this slightly
new direction.

~~~

Walking down two short gravel roads in the Montana
crisp air alone with only the bright moon as my guide I realize
how quiet my surroundings are and just how alone I am.
Shit, I did not walk along this barn before.
The gravel crunches beneath my feet as my pace picks
up both out of fear and shiver as I feel the cold Montana air
seep through my clothes and onto my now anxiously sweating
skin.
It's okay just back track, I think I just missed a turn.

The stars shine bright, more of them at once than I have ever seen, and the moon nearly bright enough to guide my walk.

Oh fuck, what happens if I can't find my way?
Oh how loaded this question really is...

She had put me in the back of the property in the most isolated and quiet cabin she had. She was the New York Times bestselling author, so I knew she had her reasons but my stubborn ass was not going to thank her that first night as I calmed down from missing a turn in the pitch black Montana night.

And I sure as hell wasn't thanking her as I laid in my bed that first of four nights attempting to journal through the deafening silence that hit my eardrums as hard as the bass at a Taylor Swift concert.

A deep breath makes tears spring to my eyes but only briefly as the clarity of my voice begins to gain strength.

These women will change my life. God, I have missed community.

And I begin to write, just a bit because tomorrow begins the first big day of finding my voice with the guidance and loving arms of Haven.

My voice, now more audible than a library whisper,

I'm here, just a bit drowned by the social media-ing, the earning a living-ing and a mission we are so desperate to accomplish.

By the third morning, she's no longer a whisper but a rather confident and renewed heart and soul-filled voice.

She's me.

With the sun shining bright, the morning air crisp with possibility and the Canadian geese as my own personal morning playlist, I walk up that gravel road alone. I am greeted by the steam rolling off the tree embraced lake and with my next step I notice her, my shadow.

My shifted shadow.

My shadow that is no longer casting my darkness ahead but rather trailing behind as if to stand in holy support.

Mustered Grace

This month, as most of us know is Pregnancy and Infant Loss Awareness Month. And, only eight days in I am working hard to hold the space to honor the paradox of the sadness and the pride I feel seeing so much talk about pregnancy and infant loss in the media and on my social media walls.

Because there is enough room for both.

Infertility, pregnancy and infant loss have lifelong costs.

We will spend the rest of our lives continually moving through the grief with whatever grace we can muster in that day.

Choosing to give ourselves permission to embrace the enigma that is defining our happy ending within the arms of lifelong loss.

It Gets Different

Every day I learn a lesson in this lifelong journey of grief.

Now a few years out of our failed infertility journey some of those lessons knock me on my ass, some push me forward and some lift me up on a firm foundation.

I am often asked,

Does it ever get better?

To which I say in complete love and loathing of the complicated gray.

It gets different.

Some days are better.

Some are brutal.

All days, in each lesson, I am shown that it gets different.

I am different; some days better, some brutal.

They Count Too

When I profusely thank such organizations as Beat Infertility, Don't Talk About the Baby and Share for including me and my story, I both hope they know how sincere I am being but also know they are probably thinking,
Of course, what is the big deal?
My words of thanks come from a place of love formed in the darkness of loss.
I have never been pregnant.
Thank God because being pregnant for me after two back surgeries and a year in a body cast would never lead to the normal celebratory leap of joy over 2 pink lines that those of us in the infertility and loss community long for.
My surrogate never achieved pregnancy with our embryos either.
And yet, there is not a National Failed Infertility Treatment Awareness Month or National IVF Embryos Count Too Awareness Month, and so the month of October's Pregnancy and Infant Loss Awareness Month is where I fall (or perhaps force my way in). Even though I can at times feel like the odd man out, left behind or the girl just beyond the outskirts of fitting in often wondering to myself,
They probably don't think I belong here. I did not lose enough. I am not enough.
That damn inner critic and scarcity, and yet, I know I am nowhere near alone.
Just as my friend over at Another Forty commented on of my last posts:
> *Having never been pregnant, though, I realize that I still have some shame related to whether or not pregnancy and infant loss awareness month applies to me. I have these pictures of our four embryos that feel like the only tangible remnant of our efforts, the closest I ever got to pregnancy. But at the end of the day I never did get there. So does it still count? I want it to desperately, and I want others to recognize it. It is such an odd thing to lose something you never really had.*

To which I replied:

Those pictures of my 8 celled babies are not only cells in a petri dish to me, never strong enough to take strong footing in a warm mother's womb, they are my babies. They count, they most definitely count. I am with you sister, it sometimes feels like there is not a place for us, but I assure you it is here. We too became mothers the day we dreamed of becoming mothers.

To you, they may simply be 8 celled embryos who were a science experiment in a sterile lab and petri dish.

To me they were growing babies, made up of Chad's athletic ability and kind heart and my red hair and passionate personality, and transferred to Michelle's loving motherly womb. My babies who never took a breath of this earth's fresh air and who I must parent from afar for the rest of my life always wondering who they might have been and who I might have been as their mother.

Tonight we will join families all over the world in the Wave of Light as we light three candles in honor of our soul scars.

And as I look at those bright flames, I will wonder if they are proud of me, wishing they were here while all in the same breath knowing all is okay.

I will also say thank you.

Thank you for including me and for remembering mothers like us.

Even In Our Longing

Never to feel the relief at the sound of your first cry.
And yet, I imagine your giggles, always.
Never to know your name.
And yet, you are known and spoken by my heart,
always.
Never to feel the warmth of your skin in my arms.
And yet, I feel you holy every day, always.
Never to know the tangible completeness; always
wondering who you might have been and who we might have
been.
And yet, trusting and knowing we are whole, even in
our longing, always.

Negotiations with a Three Year Old

As a trained and experienced therapist I know the five stages of grief well.

As a survivor of loss I'll tell you where you can stick those five stages.

Loss leaves us forever changed and not wrapped up pretty with a bow in the 5th and final stage of acceptance.

Rather, grief and loss are like handling negotiations with the average three year old; riding the waves between wild, stubborn tantrums full of attitude and affectionate cuddles sprinkled with articulated love.

Grief can feel like the dramatic threenager, and sometimes we just have to be along for the ride.

Part III

Year 3

Small and Mighty

Wherever I travel I visit the local butterfly pavilion/house/garden/sanctuary/palace, this should not be a surprise to you by now folks. My recent annual trip with my parents to Branson, Missouri always means a trip to The Butterfly Palace.

This year we only had to share the space with a handful of people on a slow day in December and of course around 1,000 butterflies. Walking around in the warm humid air, as sweat trickled down my back, I took pictures for the blog and thanked God for the miracle and beauty of the butterfly.

During the butterfly release I was blessed to meet a Butterfly Palace employee as she noticed my tattoo. Through a quick explanation of my story, honoring my babies and telling her about the meaning of butterflies to me, I made a quick connection with someone who gets it; a fellow warrior in life, a survivor of the struggle.

She soon found *Ever Upward* and commented:

I love your honesty and your transparency. I think if you were a butterfly you'd be a beautiful, delicate-yet-strong Glasswing!

And so, after a quick Google search on the Glasswing butterfly I am astonished at the home I feel in the parallels to this incredible creature.

The Glasswing butterfly has wings which are quite literally see-through. Where other butterflies have scales, the Glasswing does not. The transparent wings make it difficult to see the butterfly, at times making it appear invisible.

Not much unlike how invisible I can feel as a woman without children in our society. Often times feeling forgotten, left behind and misunderstood. I find myself fighting the urge to hustle to be seen and overwhelmed by the fear that I am invisible.

The Spanish name for the glasswing is 'espejitos'. Literally translated, this means little mirrors.

Not much unlike how much I am constantly doing the work to see myself, to work on my own insight and improve my well-being and self; in other words owning my shit. The work of self-evaluation and self-responsibility has been the only way I have dug my way out, chosen *change*, embraced all the parts of my story and defined my own happy ending.

The Glasswing is one of the strongest species of butterflies. Although it might look delicate and perhaps even powerless, it has the ability to carry nearly 40 times its own weight. It is also very fast, with the ability to fly up to eight miles per hour for short periods of time.

Not much unlike me, I am little but strongly capable. And for those who know me well, you know that I do nothing slow…ever (sometimes to my own *demise*).

And so, I guess I see a lot of myself in the Glasswing butterfly and again am in complete awe of the lessons, the connections and the miracles; of this incredible life.

And there is your biology lesson for the day ;)!

The Empty Well

Sometimes our loved ones do not have what we need, or perhaps, what we deserve.

Our work is in accepting their limitations, loving them anyways and setting boundaries if need be.

Stop going to an empty well expecting there to be water.

But, also do not be the person who stops going to the well completely, because people can change, grow and surprise us.

Instead, go to the well to enjoy the sun, the beautiful flowers and the peace you can find in yourself and in your acceptance.

And, if there is water one day, if your loved one can give you what you want, need and deserve, you can be pleasantly surprised.

Identity Theft

She sits in the chair across from me showing more of her pregnancy. Her face is filling out, her breathing becoming more and more labored and her belly growing each week as her baby gets closer to breathing this earth's fresh air.

"How is your anxiety?" I ask her with both love and accountability. "Getting any better since you passed the week of Sarah's loss?" referring to her pregnancy loss and making sure to name her baby girl.

"Maybe a little," she replies as she tries to push the tears down and away from springing to her eyes.

"There is enough room for both. Give yourself permission to feel happy and scared and anxious and sad and joyful all at the same time. Fighting any of it, or denying it, will only make the anxiety worse."

She looks at me with a look of both disbelief and peace.

Infertility and loss steals so much from us but most of us only realize how much it actually steals as life goes on.

In the fight to become parents, many of us will become shells of who we once were, knowing we can never go back to who that was.

It is the identity theft of infertility.

She's pregnant! Most would look at her like she should be fine. The treatments finally worked. She's having a baby!

Both as a survivor of infertility and a therapist who walks with clients through and after the journey, I know it is never this simple.

Infertility is lifelong, and eventually you must choose how it defines you.

No matter how your story ends up.

For me, it didn't work. Our family portrait is not complete with the 2.5 kids. The losses and costs of the infertility journey, and the loss of our three babies, are the stones I carry in my pocket every day for the rest of my life.

For some of my clients, it has ended with children, and yet, they too are left with scars for a lifetime.

The scars of the babies who never took a breath of this earth's fresh air.

The scars of the financial burdens.

The scars of the damage to their relationships.

The scars of losing themselves to the journey.

The scars of anger and bitterness.

No matter how the infertility journey ends, like anything in our lives, we choose how it leaves us. These scars leave us with plenty to be bitter about. There is also plenty to find joy and gratitude in and for.

We simply must choose it.

"Are you okay every day?" my client asks me referring to my own recovery.

"Oh gosh, not every day. But more days than not now," I reply with my usual authentic truth.

"How?"

"I fight for it, I define it and I am grateful. I was chosen to be their mother, even if only in the capacity I got them. I choose to know that God gave them to me. And for that, I am forever grateful. But in the same breath I give myself permission to also long for them and wonder always."

"A choice," said more as a statement than a question.

"Some days an easy choice, other days one that I have to fight tooth and nail through sadness and anger for. My lesson through it all has been this complicated gray. When I give myself permission to feel it all in the same breath, the longing and the gratitude, I find my life again. The awakened life in color."

"The complicated gray, huh?" she muses back both as a challenge and an acceptance.

"The damn complicated gray."

Becoming a Gift

Sitting over tea in a dimly lit coffee shop she asks, "How often do you think of them?"

I shift my eyes to notice how many moms and babies are in the bustling shop. "Every day," I respond.

"How?" she asks.

"I wonder how different our lives would be. I wonder what they would be learning and what we could be teaching them. I wonder who they would have been and who we could have been."

She looks down into her steaming cup of tea and she adjusts her body as if feeling uncomfortable in the booth. "It lasts forever doesn't it?"

"I think so."

"Does it get better?" she asks. I know she's hoping I will say that it does.

"It gets different," I respond.

I glance down at her very pregnant belly and ask what must become the most annoying question for pregnant women, "How are you feeling?"

"I'm getting tired and uncomfortable but good!" she exclaims being careful to not complain too much.

"How does it feel after everything?" I ask her no longer being able to not show her the compassionate therapist side of me.

"Being pregnant after loss is so hard," she says, barely getting the words out as her eyes fill with tears.

"I know. It can feel so impossible," I assure her with the knowing knowledge of suffering loss myself but most especially as a mental health therapist who has walked alongside many women through the infertility, loss and pregnancy after loss journey.

I lean forward and make sure to exude the love and empathy I have with her. She takes a sip of her tea and sets the cup down a bit forcefully startling both of us, "Why doesn't anyone talk about this or warn us about it?"

"I am trying to change that, I promise."

***

The only evidence I have of my three children are black and white pictures from our infertility clinic. The photos show three blobs of 8 cells; and they are my children.

My children I parent from afar.

A grief journey that many will never understand or even try to understand.

A journey that has changed my life so much I can say I am actually learning to trust it. I am honored God chose my husband and me to be their parents, if only in so much as forever wondering about them and getting that one grainy black and white picture.

Because so much has been born of them.

Without them I would not have fought my way out of darkness. Without them I would not have changed my entire life to become the incredible woman living the life I never dreamed today. Without them, my legacy would have been much different.

Because God chose me to be their mother, I found my place in His story.

Because I am their mother, I defined my own happy ending through my longing joy, in what I call the complicated gray.

The complicated gray is the muck we must walk into, the space between the happiness and the anger, the trust and the loss, the worry and the acceptance, the joy and the longing. Because when I give myself permission to feel it all, to walk into the complicated gray, life awakens in color.

And in that color I have painted a life redefined, a life of coming alive.

Alive in creativity of writing and shining my light through darkness.

Alive in creating life in monarch farming.

Alive in fighting for my joy.

Alive in advocating for self-care.

Alive in deeper and healthier relationships.

Alive in breaking the silence.

Alive in changing the conversations.

Alive in helping others.

Alive in birthing a rare kind of parenthood.

***

We sip our tea in a bit of silence. She rubs her hand over her smooth belly and I listen to the giggles of the babies and their moms enjoying a snack at the coffee shop.

"You are a gift," she finally breaks the silence.

"I have become a gift because of them."

Loving Well and Fully

I have found a special love, and talent for those in the battle of secondary infertility and those in the midst of pregnancy after loss.

The other day I had an aha with a client coping with pregnancy after loss. One of the biggest misconceptions of the trying to conceive, infertility and loss community is that a healthy pregnancy is our cure all. I see some of the hardest struggle during this time, which if you think about it, is not that surprising. We've already had the worst case scenario happen, we already know that not everything always turns out. A healthy pregnancy, although amazing and happy, is also filled with anxiety, worry and, if we aren't careful, all consuming fear.

What I am especially seeing in my office is the difficulty for mom to allow herself to attach and fully love the growing baby in her belly, "Because what if it isn't okay? What if I lose it?"

To which I say, "Your children before this, although you may have never had the blessing to meet them, made you the mother you are today. You love this baby well because of them. You love this baby fully in honor of the ones who made you a mother to begin with."

The complicated gray of afraid and brave all at once my fellow warriors, loving well and loving fully is what our children deserve, it is also what we deserve.

The Goosebumps of Knowing Awe

The email comes through with the subject line of #MoreThan1in8 and my heart skips a beat.

The social media notification comes through with the brave words and beautiful faces of someone breaking the silence and I'm overcome with goosebumps in knowing awe.

The knowing awe of the power of telling our stories.

The knowing awe of the freedom of owning stories.

The knowing awe of the world changing.

In one week I have had 29 people share their stories of thriving through and thereafter infertility along with their bright shining faces. In the next two weeks I hope and pray that number jumps to no less than 100.

Because I want more from us and for us. It is my #startasking I suppose.

Even if you are not comfortable, now or ever, to share your infertility story publicly on social media, I would be appreciative if you would at least share the project. More than that I would be honored if you would share your story and show your face with me privately via email. I am not publicly posting the stories. I am however going to use our faces, the images of thriving through and after infertility, for a project during National Infertility Awareness Week. But your photo may not necessarily be identifiable, as it will be very, very small. Too public for you even still? Then please share your story with me and a photo of the hobby, the pets, the books that are helping you thrive through and after your infertility journey. Or if you think I'm crazy and this will never work, I'll just take those thoughts, prayers and lots of magic that this project can provide some of us the outlet to tell our stories.

But still, I beg you, break your silence in a way that honors your truth and changes your life and the world.

We cannot want more from our loved ones and our society unless we tell our stories. We must ask for what we want and need, and we must educate if we are going to get the understanding and compassion we all so desperately need through and after this journey. No need for the public blog or social media posts or publishing the book, but please, speak your story to someone who loves you, to someone you trust.

I think, speaking our truth and owning our stories, is one of the only ways we will get out of this alive and well.

Receiving the Revealed Dream

Every message I get, every review posted, every thank you received has been tucked away into the depths of my soul.

They are the reminders of how I mother, of how I honor my babies and they are the reminders I desperately need along this journey of breaking the silence of infertility and getting people to hear the healthy messages of *Ever Upward*.

This past Saturday, the closing day of National Infertility Awareness Week (NIAW), in the exhaustion of working three jobs without an assistant, I was gifted magic.

Despite my weary heart from the hard work of my #MoreThan1in8 project, God knew my NIAW wasn't finished when He presented me with my first big speaking engagement. With only a few days notice I was asked to tell my story at the Gateway to Parenthood conference put on by the Missouri Center for Reproductive Medicine.

After two years of the constant marketing of *Ever Upward* with what at times feels like no return, there was no way I could say no.

What I did not realize is that I was saying yes to me.

Waking up before the crack of dawn on a Saturday after the busiest week of my career was only saved by my curled hair, cute navy dress, heels, and of course, my Plexus and coffee.

Sitting at the table with Chad and my mom as people began to mill around I was taken aback when a tall woman with dark hair approached my table right away.

"Justine?" she said.

I stood up and reached out my hand, "Yes, I'm Justine Froelker."

"Hi, I'm Jen Myers from Y98 (aka our keynote speaker for the day). I follow you on Twitter and had to meet you."

My heart skips a beat as I force myself to take a deep breath but there is no calming down the excitement that she had to meet me?

"Oh, hi! It is so nice to meet you," I reply. "Thank you so much for using your huge platform to continue to speak about your infertility journey and losses. We need voices like yours."

She shakes her head, "Thank you, for the work you are doing."

We go on to bitch as fellow warriors about how brutal this journey is and how difficult her PCOS diagnosis has been.

When she walks away, I sit down and look at Chad and my mom with eyes wide in star struck gratitude, "Well, that was amazing!"

The first few hours we man my table as most people walk right by us without stopping. Which I can't blame them for, I didn't have any sign ups, free candy or massages to give away, just bookmarks with my wise words and my beautiful breakaway monarch from the book cover and my smile. Most of the attendees of the conference hadn't even realized they each had a copy of my book in their gift bag.

Until, they started reading.

"My husband has been reading your book all morning as I've been wondering around the tables, he can't put it down. He just told me how good it is."

Eventually, they began to trickle in for me to sign their copies.

I was supposed to speak at 11. As I was calming myself with deep breaths and rehearsing in my head, one of my now friends and volunteers asked me, "Would you try it again?"

"No, we wouldn't," I replied not sure of what she was really trying to get at.

"Really?"

"Well when the money is gone, it's gone. And, when you've reached a place of acceptance, albeit with forever longing and sadness, it is still acceptance."

"What if you won the free round giveaway today? Would you try again then?"

I was very much taken aback by this question but I knew my answer right away, "No, we are done."

Just as we are not signing up for the costs and struggles of the adoption journey, we are finished with the costs and the struggles of the infertility journey.

We did not get what we wanted, hoped for, dreamed of and paid for but we are done, we know our enoughs and everythings. And, I am okay with that, complicated gray of longing joy and all.

At 11:30 it was finally my turn to speak.

I hadn't prepared a ton. Frankly, I was too exhausted to prepare my talk after the grueling week of NIAW. For the first time, maybe in this whole journey I trusted.

God put this in my life, He would take care of it.

I took the microphone and I spoke. I taught. I loved.

I was myself.

I delivered one of the best talks of my life, because it was my story and my messages. And, I know both are needed and help myself and others.

And. It. Felt. Great.

He has finally revealed my dream to me in a way I can understand, an answered prayer for sure.

It wasn't until people came to thank me, that I realized just how much people in our community need these messages.

A husband through tears, "Thank you. You made me feel for the first time in three years. This has been so hard."

A woman with her friend, "Thank you for being the only person to get up there and say that sometimes this doesn't work and you can still be okay. Thank you for having the courage to speak anyway, we need to hear those stories too."

One of the infertility clinic's patient coordinators, "I'd like to buy your book. I've had several patients tell me how great your talk was and that I have to read your book."

A couple, "Thank you so much for all the resources, we've already downloaded some of the things you talked about. We're going to do the gratitude journals too!"

Another couple, "Thank you for getting it and for still speaking."

Another woman, "Thank you for honoring and speaking about the struggle."

As the emails trickle in as these hundreds of people finish my book, I am allowing myself to receive this amazing gift while also keeping the grief, shame and scarcity at bay.

Because, I am oh so grateful.

Grateful I was chosen to be their mother. Grateful for this life He has written for me.

Grateful I am defining my ever upward within it.

Seeing Me

I sat at a table surrounded by five other women I've known for years but hadn't seen in quite some time. There was wine being shared, except by the few who were pregnant, and a basket of forbidden (well to me) gluten with hand whipped butter being passed around the table.

I took a long sip of my red wine before taking the warm bread and smothering the butter onto it before taking a bite into a version of heaven to me.

I had come in with no expectations, yet was prepared to struggle a bit that night with a few pregnant bellies and the only one at the table who is not a traditional mother. But it had been some time since I had seen everyone and even though it was not kids I had to share about I still have an interesting life to share.

There was laughter, baby tips and birth stories.

There was not one single inquiry for me.

Not one.

I feel invisible a lot, especially marketing a book about infertility and loss. I feel invisible in our society a lot as the woman who can't have kids, where many times I am quite literally the only one everywhere I go.

Never have I felt more invisible than at that dinner table despite being surrounded by old friends. I breathed deep, engaged in the conversation and clasped my hands beneath the tablecloth harder and harder as if the pressure between my hands kept the tears from pouring down my face.

By the time I got home I was inconsolable.

I texted one of my other mom friends, "Thank you for seeing me, for always doing your best to make sure I don't feel invisible as the only one without kids. You have no idea how much that helps me survive this world."

Chad tried his best to console me as I tried to contain myself, he said, "You can cry".

He could tell I felt stupid and frustrated but there was no holding in these kinds of sobs, "It's not fair, you hardly ever have to deal with this."

He forced me into a hug and said, "You're right, guys don't talk about their kids nonstop."

He held me tighter and between sobs I managed to get out, "I will have to deal with this for the rest of my life."

As a therapist, hell as a human, I work hard to make sure every single person I am around feels seen, known and loved in my presence. Thriving after infertility without my own children has only strengthened this quality of mine.

Because I feel invisible almost all of the time.

It's been some time since that dinner, the work I have done the last several years helps me to know that this sense of being invisible is not my truth. It also helped going into National Infertility Awareness Week and my #MoreThan1in8 project and connecting with so many of my fellow warriors. But, it was scary knowing the dreaded Mother's Day was just around the corner.

The day of what feels like true disappearance from this world for a woman like me.

But this year, Mother's Day was different, for a couple of reasons.

1.   I reclaimed the day by giving myself permission to celebrate it myself.

2.   I felt more seen and loved well through it than ever before.

I received cards in the mail, texts and gifts from friends and more Facebook messages than I ever imagined. Many of these things coming from people who I never even realized were watching my journey at all, let alone cared about it.

I was a mother seen.

Because I speak my truth and own my story, sometimes to the dismay, disapproval and discernment of others, there is no choice but to know I exist.

I know my story is sad, I know it makes you uncomfortable and I know some wish I'd just stop already.

What I know now, several years into thriving, is that your denial, or perception, of my story does not change my truth.

I am seen. I am known. I am loved.

I am helping.

I am helping because I will make sure you feel seen, known and loved too.

A Strawberry Shortcake Bandage

Her scraped up knee is bright red with fresh blood. Plump tears roll down her rosy cheeks.

"Okay, ready? It is going to burn but mama will blow on it to help."

"Okay," she gets out in the midst of a sob.

I pour the clear peroxide over the freshly scraped up knee so rightfully and bravely earned from her first go around without training wheels. The familiar white bubbles appear as her leg jumps out of reflex and an audible whine escapes her mouth.

"Okay, blow on it with me," I coax her.

We both gently blow a steady stream of what has to feel like healing cool air onto the foaming and now clean injury.

"How's that?'

"Better," she musters through the slightest of smirks.

We sing a song while we wait for the boo boo to air dry.

"My Little Pony or Strawberry Shortcake bandage?" I ask.

"Strawberry," she answers with the faintest little girl accent.

That's my girl, I think back to my own Strawberry Shortcake curtains and bedding as a kid her age.

I gently place the pink and red bandage over the scrape.

"Kiss?"

"Yes."

The simplest of moments between a mother and a daughter. A moment I am sure most parents never give a second thought to. For me, a moment in my forever longing and wondering imagination. Yet, I got some semblance of it this weekend when one of my clients texted me for help. She was off visiting where she is going to continue her college education far, far away from the city limits of St. Louis and in the mountains where she spent the last couple of days hiking much to the chagrin of her heels.

A picture of the biggest blister I have ever seen came through on my phone with a message of, "Please tell me what to do. Do I clean it? Cover it? Help. Please."

Not the normal text I get as a mental health therapist, yet one I wasn't surprised by.

I talked her through cleaning her blisters and taking care of them but at first forgot to tell her about blowing on the foaming peroxide! My self-talk was not much unlike what I hear in my office from mothers who hardly ever give themselves credit for the brilliant jobs they are doing, Crap! God, I suck.

I circled back and let her know to blow on the bubbles to help with the sting. I then told her that I was sorry she was never taught this growing up and that she deserved better. Her mother died when she was young and she grew up without a mother like figure to teach her these kinds of things.

And, I am growing old without my own children to teach them to.

God's plan in something as simple as a boo boo.

Much of what we do as therapists is re-parenting our clients. I teach, I coach, I push, I hold space for healing, I keep accountable and I deeply care. Actually, this is also what I do if you are my friend or family. It is kind of impossible to shut off.

It was there before the infertility journey. Only, made stronger by becoming a mother to my three. And, something I am thankful for every single day.

The bossy, pushy, loving mother I am. The mother they made me. The mother armed with the breath of healing and a Strawberry Shortcake bandage.

The Permission of And

I stand on my brick patio looking up at the churning sky. My lush butterfly gardens, all four of them, surround me with all the shades of green you can imagine and the sweetest scents to ever fill my nose.

I force the deep breath in through my nose in an attempt to not allow the sobs to escape and tears to roll.

I look up, *God* I need something. Take this away if it isn't for Your good or Your plan. Give me something, show me what I need to keep going, that I am on the right track. Please give me the strength either way.

Three pleads. Three requests.

Three.

And, there they are again.

I release the deep breath from my mouth which only seems to give permission for the tears to come.

I breath in again, breathing in how much my soul longs for my three, Have you forgotten me?

I make myself pause with my exhale; stopping to listen.

The birds are chirping and the wind is blowing through my milkweed plants and all the trees.

In the breath of the wind and churning of the sky I hear, I am here child. I've got it. I am good. Trust me.

I feel a new and slight sense of peace and my lingering frustration. Once again, I am reminded of the complicated gray I feel everyday without my children here on earth.

The complicated gray of the longing joy and the childless mother.

With eyes and heart wide open to receive and the courage to ask, the next two weeks He fills my life with example after example of the complicated gray. As if He is saying, Make the time, this is your path, write it, share it, shine it.

The client who is about to deliver her sons after years of trying; feeling happy and scared.

My team who battles the fear of what others think and their belief and bravery to help others and share something they believe in.

The client who loves and must let go of people she really cares about.

The reader who is finally pregnant after years of trying only to realize her fear is stealing her joy.

The muck between knowing we are worthy, lovable, enough and the old stories our head tells us that we aren't.

The acquaintance who desperately wants and needs to make a change in her life and feels comfortable even if it is in her known misery.

The client who is very early in a pregnancy after a miscarriage and a stillbirth, feeling the pull to protect the memory of her sons while also loving and hoping for this new baby.

My pride in a growing business and the frustration in it not happening fast enough.

All of the complicated gray and what I am learning is my gift for this world.

Because the complicated gray is the permission to change the but to an and.

Giving ourselves permission to feel it all, all at the same time; the anger and acceptance, the joy and the longing, the fear and the hope.

The permission to walk into the muck of the gray between the certainties of life; allowing ourselves to hold both truths, as difficult and uncomfortable as that is, we will awaken to life in color.

The anxious hope. The doubting worth. The frustrated belief. The boundaried love. The yearning acceptance.

The longing joy as the childless mother.

So, I will continue to fight for this next book because it is needed, I see the power in it every day in my life and He seems to be reminding me of it more and more.

Thank you for your patience as I continue my advocacy work, my jobs that actually pay the bills and working on the follow up to *Ever Upward*. And, I'll take whatever prayers, positive sparkles, love and shares/tweets/likes you've got.

Four

The three of you would have turned four this year.
Four.
The year of becoming little people. The terrible language barriers and potty training of the 2's out of the way and the dramatics of the 3's in our past.
Four.
The years I have spent wondering of you every day, feeling you always and wandering this earth with pieces of my soul tethered to heaven.

I've been told to write a letter to you a few times and for quite some time. But, it wasn't until I asked one of my warrior mamas to write her babies a letter in hopes of her finding some clarity and healing, even within the uncertain darkness of infertility, that I realized you deserved and I need my words.

I could write of how much I miss you and yet feel like I never had you. The weeks of synthetic hormones to retrieve you, the five days to only hear about your growth in a phone call from the infertility clinic and the gut wrenching two weeks of praying and hoping you would stick in her warm uterus. All to end in a one minute phone call with the words, "She's not pregnant." Years of trying, tens of thousands of dollars spent and lifelong dreams crushed in a phone call telling me our relationship was over before I even got to meet you.

I was not a mother.

And, I believed that for a long while.

It was dark, there were tears, a lot of anger and a sense of self that disappeared behind never being seen.

I could write of all my wonderings. Would you have had my freckles or your dad's blonde curls? Would you have been spunky like me or stoic like him? Would I have handled the poop and he the puke? What books would have been your favorite in your nighttime routine? What kind of grandparents would they have been? I could fill the biggest library on earth with my wonderings of the last four years, let alone of the lifetime of wonderings ahead of me.

I am a mother.

I worry, I wonder, I question, I doubt, I love.

Even if only from afar.

I could write how forgotten you and my motherhood are most days. No one speaks of you, some even say you don't count. Many aren't sure what to ask me or how to relate to me; a childless mother, I am often the only one everywhere I go.

The invisible mother.

The one without the happy ending.

Yet, only through you have I fought for, found and created my own happy ending of thriving.

What I hope you know is how loved and wanted you are and were.

I hope I make you proud.

I hope every day you are honored in my work, my words, and especially, my love.

I have learned God gifted you to me, even if only for a whisper of time, as you were always His to begin with. I am blessed He chose me as your mother, it is the best gift I have ever received.

In the lifelong absence and the daily presence of you, I have found me.

It is because of you I notice every sunset and sunrise, see beauty in pain, feel with my whole being, believe in the unseen, give more than I ever have, seek the unknown, laugh with childlike wonder, walk with curiosity and have more gratitude for it all than ever before.

It is because of you I love harder and better.

Four.

I love you always.

Four.

Thank you, my loves.

mom

A Story the World Isn't Ready For... Yet

I sit at the dining room table. The slightest glimmer of the rising sun brightening the sky outside the floor to ceiling window as I take the first drink of my yummy, albeit nutritious, breakfast smoothie. My usual songs of rising playing and my coloring journal in front of me. Oftentimes my morning writing turns into written prayers, as if talking to Him helps to clear my head while also making it all the more real.

The work I am doing. The words I am speaking. The fight I am fighting.

I know He is listening, and yet I often have to remind myself I am not alone in this.

When suddenly I am surprised by the words I am writing, my own words, in the chosen color of pink for today, *Why Lord did you write this story for me if you aren't going to give people the ears and hearts to hear it?*

As soon as I see the sentence, the prayer, it does not take but a half breath for the next sentence to come out of my hand, *Give ears to the earless.*

I close my eyes as an exasperated breath escapes my lips, damn it.

Yep, I curse, even when I talk to Him. He knows I am thinking it anyways. And, guess what? He loves me anyway.

Please God, help me to find a way to do this. I pray for clarity, creativity and courage to create the openness...

Perception may be that I am uber successful, the emails I get each week thanking me for my work and also asking to take me to lunch to learn from me speak to this. And yet, most days I feel as if I am jumping up and down, waving my arms desperately and screaming, "Does anyone see me? Can anyone hear?"

I have come to realize I am in the business of the invisible unspoken; I speak my life into a world of people who don't want to hear my story, in fact some of them actively deny it.

Let's just start with therapy. The stigma is changing as people begin to not only admit but boast that they see a great therapist and you should too. Yet, mental illness is widely misunderstood by both the general public and I am finding even more so by the medical community; let alone, that happiness is a choice and takes intentional daily work. I am a therapist. People love my resources, my education and inspiration. Yet, they struggle, and sometimes even refuse, to do the damn work themselves.

Then we've got my side gig in network marketing with a supplement company that I am very proud of, whose products have changed my life and an industry I love more and more each day. The misconceptions on network marketing and supplementation are endless. People question my motives, products and the industry daily. When all I am trying to do is help myself and others find freedom in their health and finances. Rather, than open up to a different way, what I think is a better way, many choose to stay in their known misery (not much unlike my daily work as a therapist).

Finally, my purpose and calling here on earth; my motherhood, although most won't call it that. My story scares most people, I am the epitome of life not turning out how you planned, hoped, dreamed or paid for. I am the worst case scenario: tried to have kids, paid a lot of money to have kids and ended the journey without them.

I am childless and a mother.

I am the case who lowers the infertility clinics statistics because I did not get the baby and I am the therapist who is helping women thrive through and after this journey no matter what they get. Because despite what the media and the average clinic wants you to believe, not all of us end up with babies; yet there are many versions of the happy ending, I promise.

I am the infertility community's black sheep and one of the hardest working advocates for anyone no matter where they are in the journey. I know my narrative scares the shit out of most and yet it is my scary story, the permission to speak the unspoken and to say enough that helps so many thrive no matter what they get in life.

I am the general society's unacknowledged unsuccess story and a change maker, even if only on the tiniest of scales. People want the story of someone who never gave up and got the traditional happy ending. When in reality those stories are actually few and far between because none of us get out of this life without having to redefine something and choosing to thrive thereafter. My truth is about thriving when life did not turn out, and despite what is shared in the media, or even in my own community, I have one hell of a happy ending. I fight for it, create it and receive it every day.

I was made the mother I am to teach and model it for you.

Now sitting on my orange couch flanked by three little dogs, I take a sip of my steaming decaf coffee. I set the timer on my phone for five minutes for my creative writing which begins as a continuation of my earlier written prayers. My handwriting slows down and clears up after I write again, why give me this story if no one is ready to hear it?

Because, my child, it is not about you, it is about them. It is about Me. Therefore go out and love like Me. Walking in the grace and the mess of truth in love and the complicated gray. I promise, you were made for such a time as this and they are listening.

Epilogue

There you have it.

Three years of flawed and continually evolving writing.

I hope you find your *me too* in my journey.

I hope shining my light helps you to shine your light out of the darkness.

And, I hope you choose to define your own happy ending and to rise ever upward.

I am not sure yet what God's plan is for *Ever Upward*. For the first time in my life I can say I have completely handed it over to Him. Together, with Him, I will continue to do the work to release my pain so that I can help even more people and honor my three.

My next step in this journey is the release of my next book, *The Complicated Gray*, in the Fall of 2017. *The Complicated Gray* is completely different than *Ever Upward* and something I am proud of and so excited to share. It is, quite possibly, one of the most important lessons I've learned from this journey, and in the least, filled with some great stories.

Please make sure to follow at www.everupward.org for updates. Thank you so much for reading.

Thank you, especially, for seeing me.

Justine

Made in the USA
Middletown, DE
02 November 2019

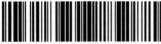

77672666R00099